SLIDE INTERPRETATION IN POSTGRADUATE MEDICINE

P. S. PARFREY and J. CUNNINGHAM

Lecturers in Medicine, The London Hospital, UK

Oxford Melbourne Delhi

OXFORD UNIVERSITY PRESS

Oxford University Press, Walton Street, Oxford OX2 6DP

London   Glasgow   New York   Toronto
Delhi   Bombay   Calcutta   Madras   Karachi
Kuala Lumpur   Singapore   Hong Kong   Tokyo
Nairobi   Dar es Salaam   Cape Town
Melbourne   Auckland

and associated companies in
Beirut   Berlin   Ibadan   Mexico City   Nicosia

OXFORD *is a trademark of Oxford University Press*

© *P. S. Parfrey and J. Cunningham 1980*

First published 1980
Reprinted 1983

British Library Cataloguing in Publication Data
Parfrey, P S
Slide interpretation in postgraduate
medicine.—(Oxford medical publications).
1. Symptomatology
I. Title   II. Cunningham, J   III. Series
616'.0022'2   RC69   80-40694
ISBN *0–19–261282–4*

Typeset in Hong Kong by
Asco Trade Typesetting Ltd.
Printed in Hong Kong by
Hip Shing Offset Printing Factory

9.95

OXFORD MEDICAL PUBLICATIONS

SLIDE INTERPETATION
IN POSTGRADUATE
MEDICINE

Acknowledgements

This book has been written as a result of our experience in teaching MRCP candidates in the London Hospital, where the vast majority of the slides reproduced here originated. In particular we thank Professor J. M. Ledingham, Dr F. J. Goodwin, and Dr M. G. Molloy for permission to use their slides. We are also indebted to Ms Alison Langton of Oxford University Press, who got this project off the ground and then kept it going, and Mrs B. Winehouse for precise and protective secretarial assistance.

Contents

Introduction

Undergraduate and postgraduate examinations have changed in format during the past decade, less emphasis being placed on essay questions and more emphasis on multiple choice and data interpretation questions. In some postgraduate examinations, especially the Membership of the Royal College of Physicians' diploma, slides have been introduced to test interpretation of clinical signs and of clinical problems. This book has been written because examination success is related in part to familiarity with the kind of questions set. We have produced both slides and questions so that candidates for postgraduate medical examinations may practise their approach to slide interpretation and form an idea of the type of knowledge required to pass the examination.

In the MRCP diploma the slide section of the examination consists of 20 slides with relevant questions, answers to which must be written within two minutes. Each question has one or two stems (occasionally three). Sometimes a clue is given with the question to help interpret the slide, especially when more than one correct interpretation could be made of the slide. It is important to look carefully at all parts of the slide, although the abnormality is very likely to be in the centre. When the abnormality has been identified, the candidate should look again at the rest of the slide. Some of the questions we ask in this book are a little more difficult than those asked in MRCP, but we have presented both slides and questions as they would be in MRCP. We have reproduced fewer radiographs than have been presented in MRCP recently, the ratio of radiographs to physical signs having been about 1:2. Occasionally, slides of blood films and pathology specimens have also been shown.

Five papers, containing 20 questions each, are presented in this book. It is hoped that candidates will use each paper as a mock examination. Answers with a relevant discussion are given at the end of each paper. The amount of information given in the answers is not uniform or comprehensive. Readers should look up doubtful points in a textbook where they are treated more fully. (See list of reference textbooks.)

PAPER 1

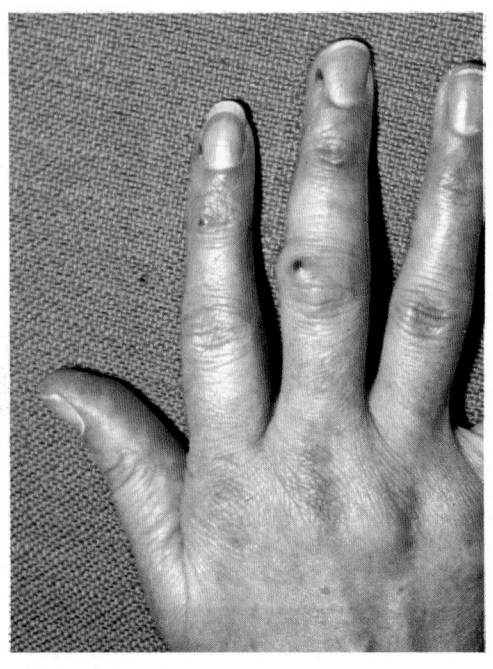

Q 1.1   (a) Name three abnormal physical signs.

(b) What is the most likely diagnosis?

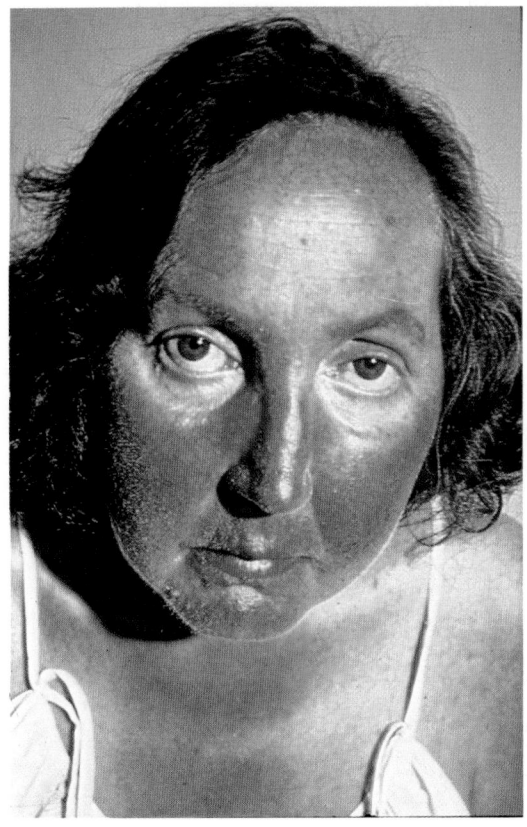

Q 1.2   This woman complains of diarrhoea of one year's duration.

(a) What is the diagnosis?

(b) Name three symptoms commonly associated with this condition.

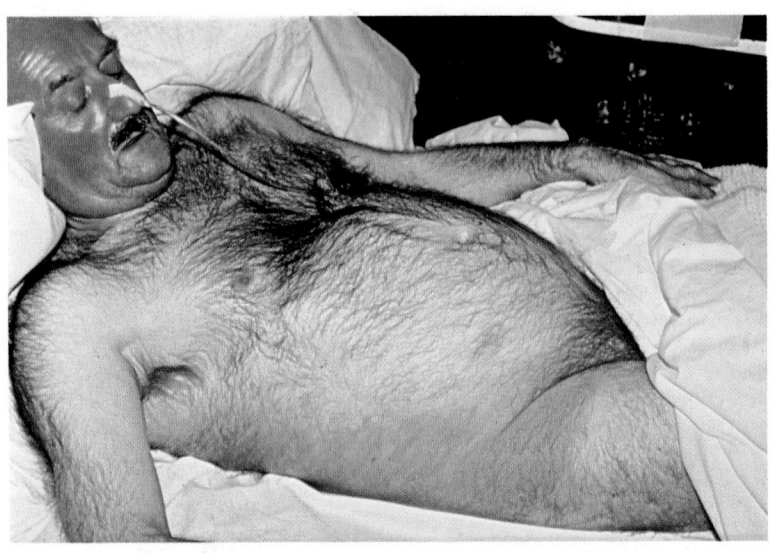

Q 1.3   This patient presented with severe abdominal pain and is in shock.

(a) Name the abnormal physical sign on this slide.

(b) What is the most likely diagnosis?

(c) What are the two most important factors predisposing to this disorder?

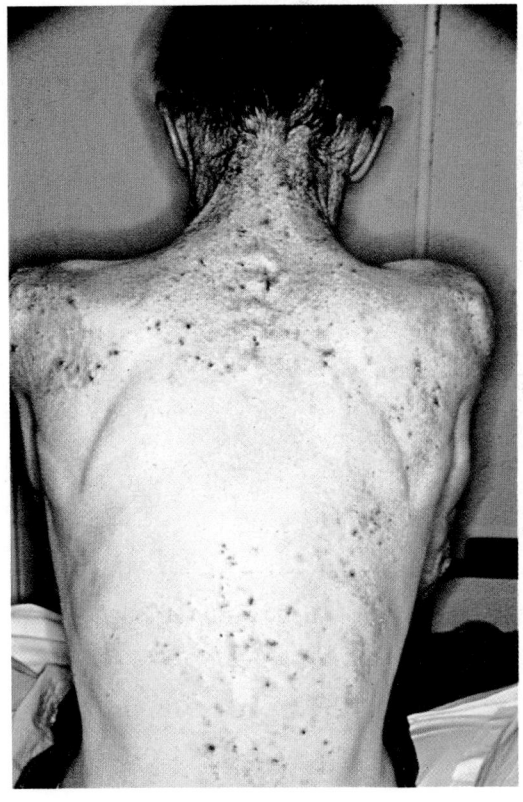

Q 1.4   This patient complains of intense pruritus.

(a) What drug will usually relieve the pruritus?

(b) What is the characteristic immunofluorescence finding on skin biopsy in this disorder?

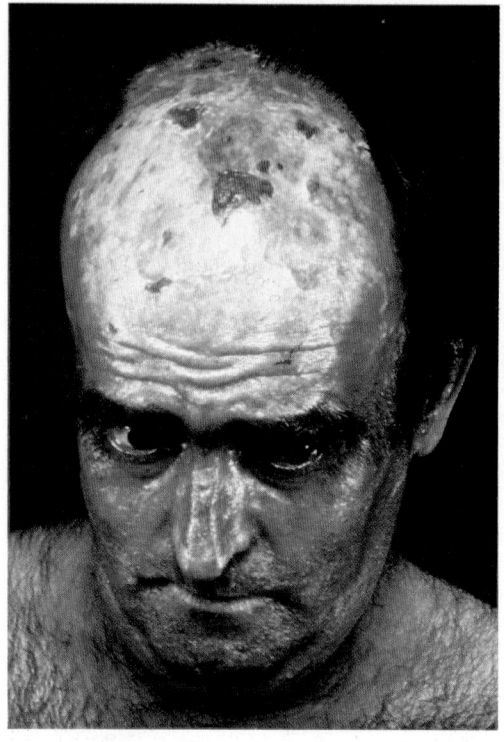

Q 1.5   This patient has chronic liver disease and developed blisters on his
head and hands while on summer holidays.

What is the most likely diagnosis?

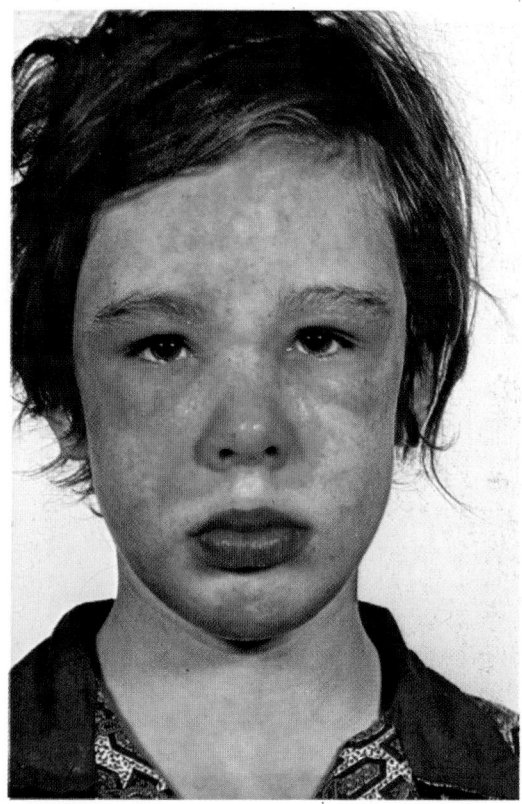

Q 1.6   This patient felt weak and was referred to out-patients for investigation of dysphagia.

    (a) What is the diagnosis?

    (b) What three investigations would you do to confirm your diagnosis?

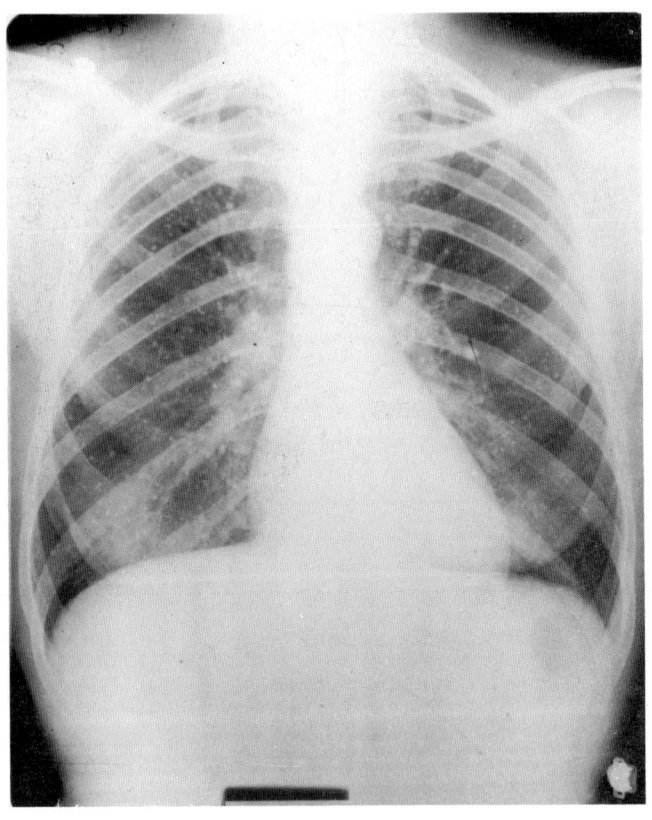

Q 1.7   A 40-year-old man developed a rash and four days later became dyspnoeic. This chest X-ray was taken three years later.

(a) What abnormality is shown on the chest X-ray?

(b) What is the most likely diagnosis?

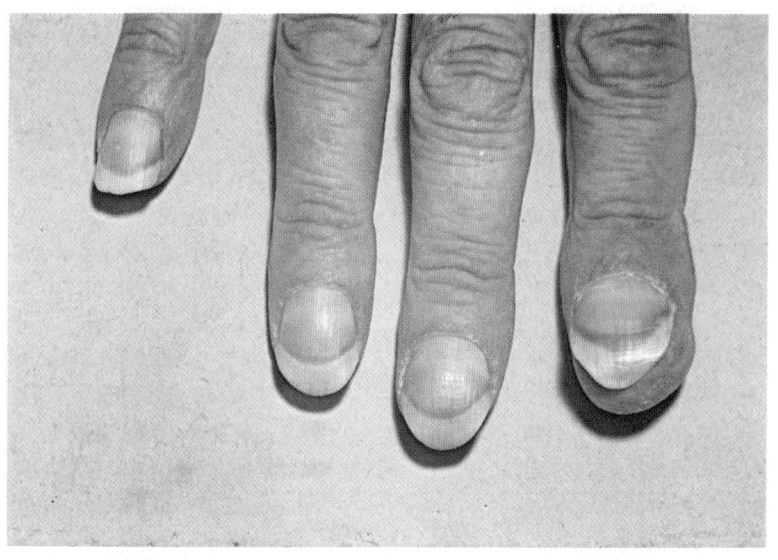

Q 1.8   This patient has end-stage renal failure.

Name two abnormal physical signs.

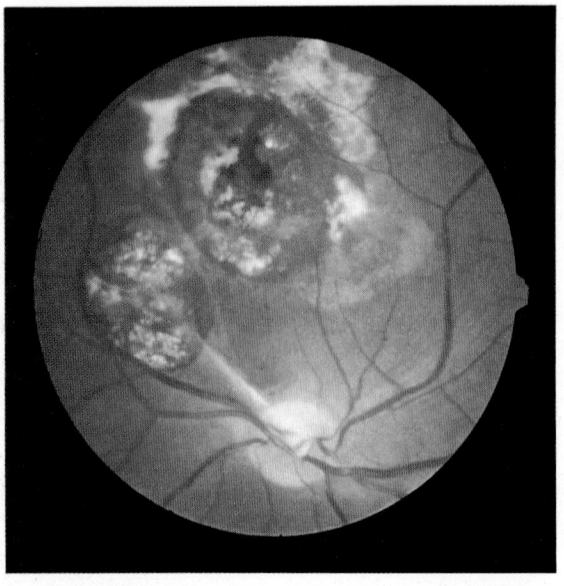

Q 1.9   What is the most likely cause of this lesion?

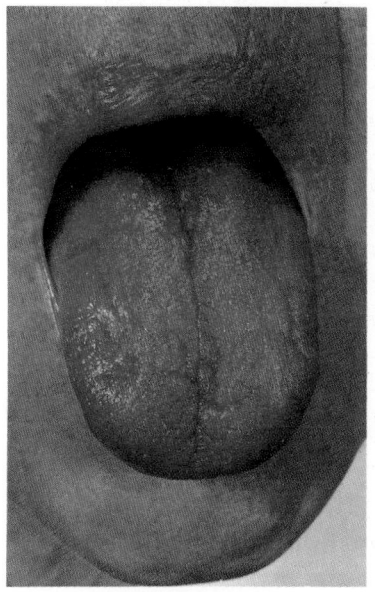 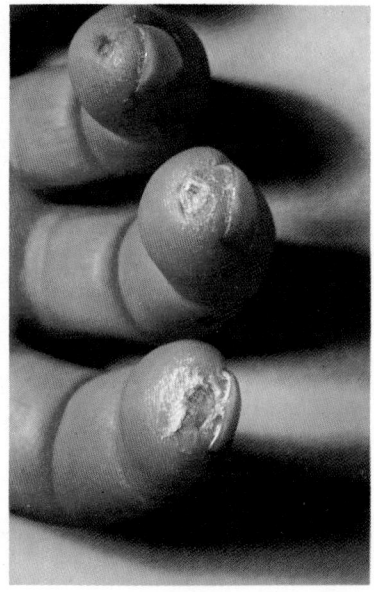

Q 1.10 These two slides are of the same patient who complained of painful eyes for two months.

(a) What is the most likely diagnosis?

(b) What test would you do to confirm the cause of this patient's sore eyes?

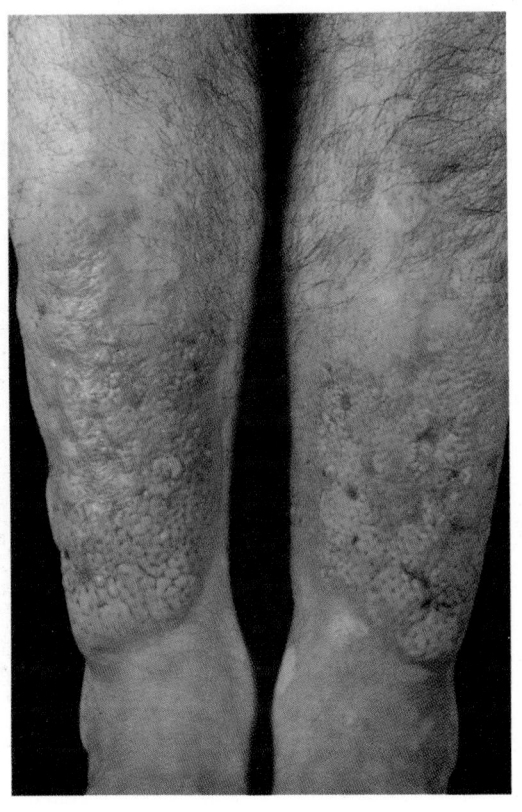

Q 1.11   (a) Name two abnormal physical signs and

(b) a serological test with which this sign is characteristically associated.

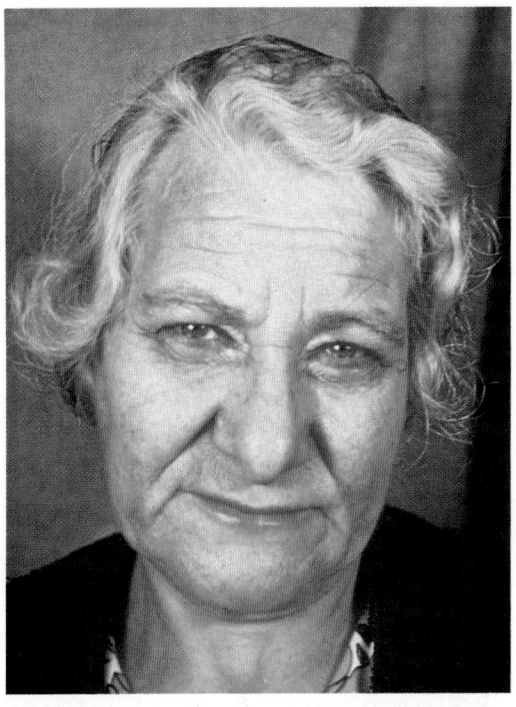

Q 1.12   This patient has pruritis.

(a) Name the abnormal physical sign.

(b) What is the most likely diagnosis?

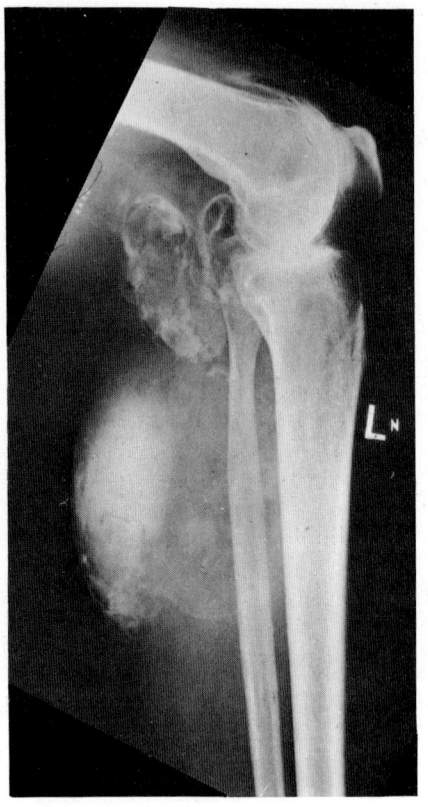

Q 1.13 This patient has rheumatoid arthritis.

(a) What is the abnormality visible on this X-ray?

(b) What may be the consequence of this abnormality?

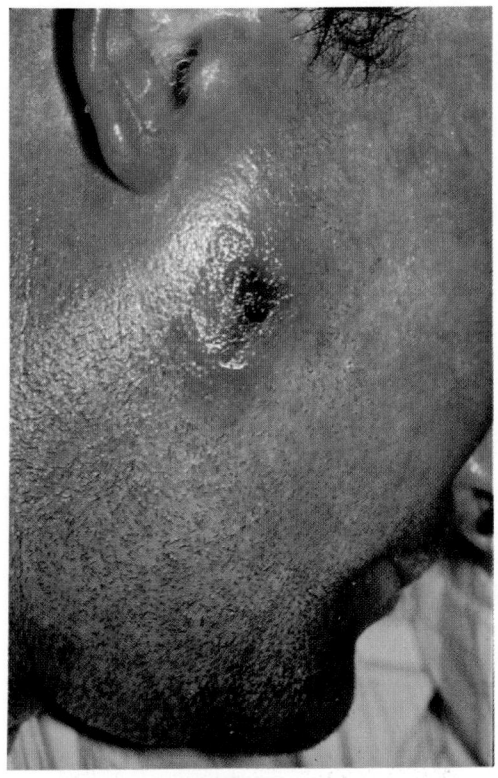

Q 1.14   This lesion is pruritic and not very tender. There is mild regional lymphadenopathy.

(a) How did this patient acquire this lesion?

(b) How would you treat this problem?

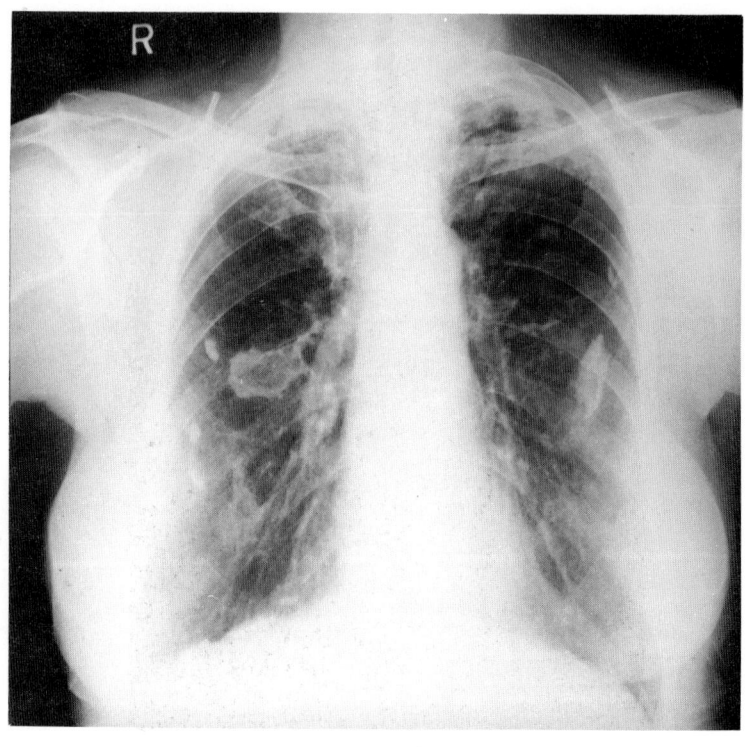

Q 1.15   (a) What is the diagnosis?

(b) What are the two most likely causes of death?

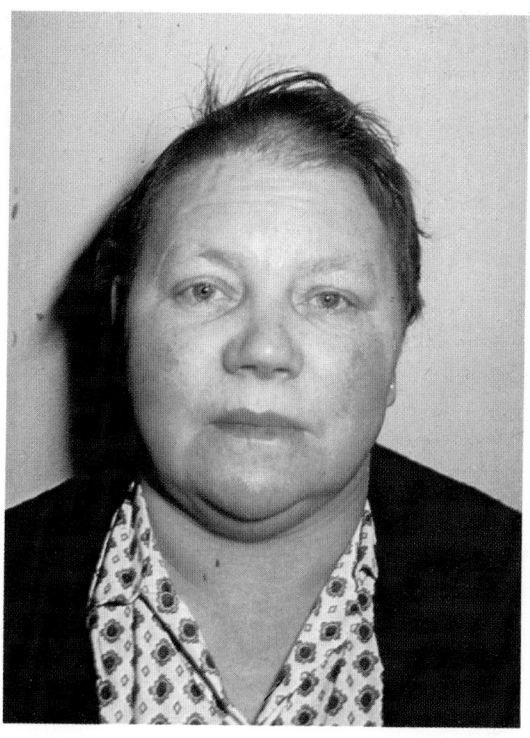

Q 1.16   This patient is anaemic.

    (a) Name three possible causes of the anaemia.

    (b) Name two abnormalities which are likely to be seen on the ECG of this patient.

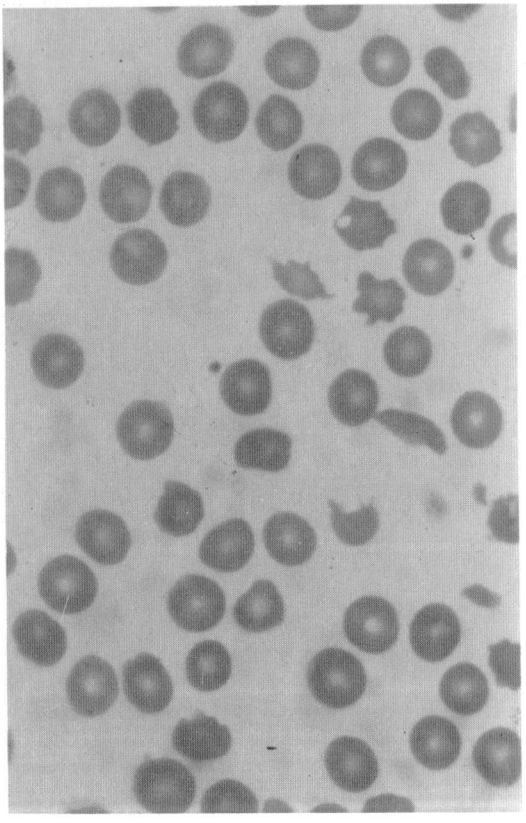

Q 1.17   (a) Name two abnormal cells visible on this blood film.

(b) Name four important causes of this picture.

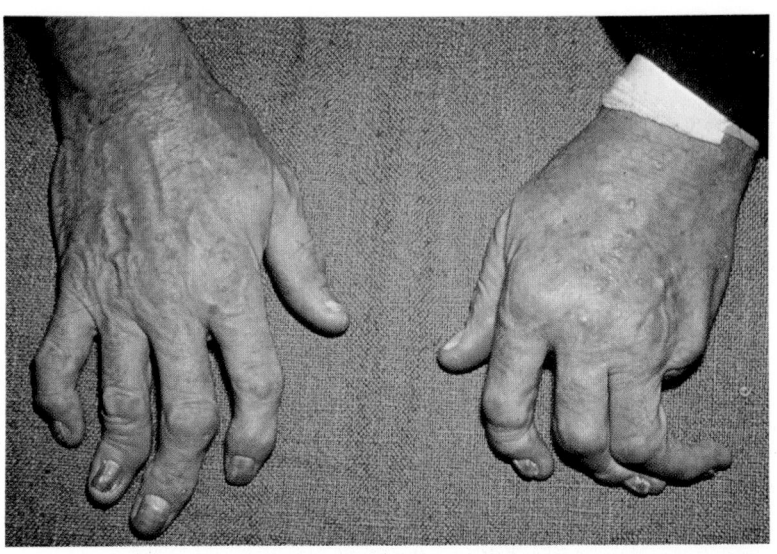

Q 1.18   (a) Name three abnormal physical signs.

              (b) What will the X-ray of the hands reveal?

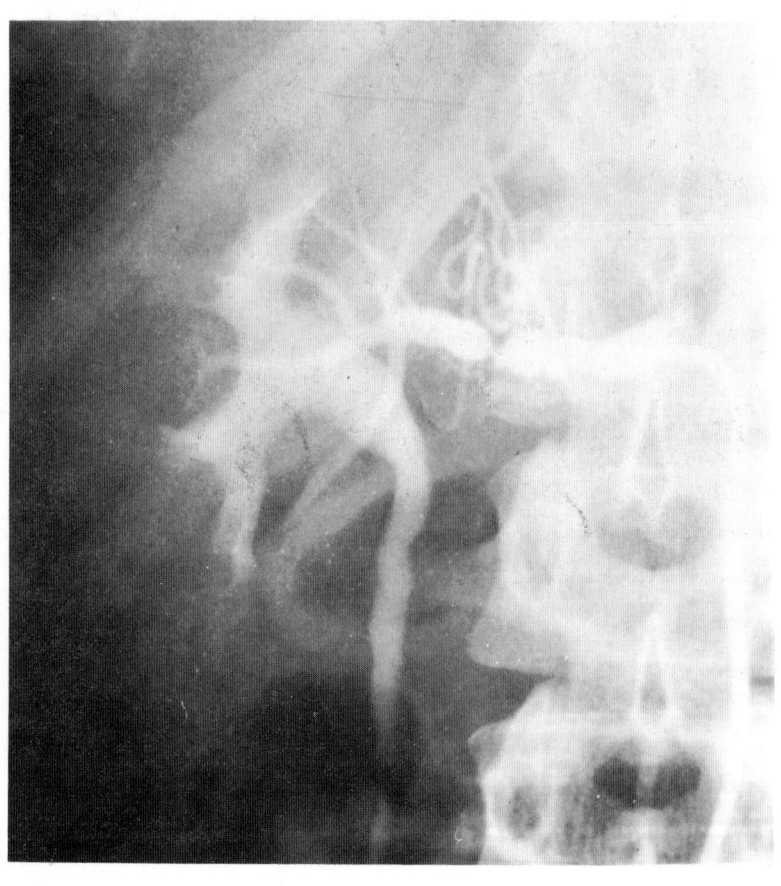

Q 1.19 Name three abnormalities which may be visible on IVP of this patient.

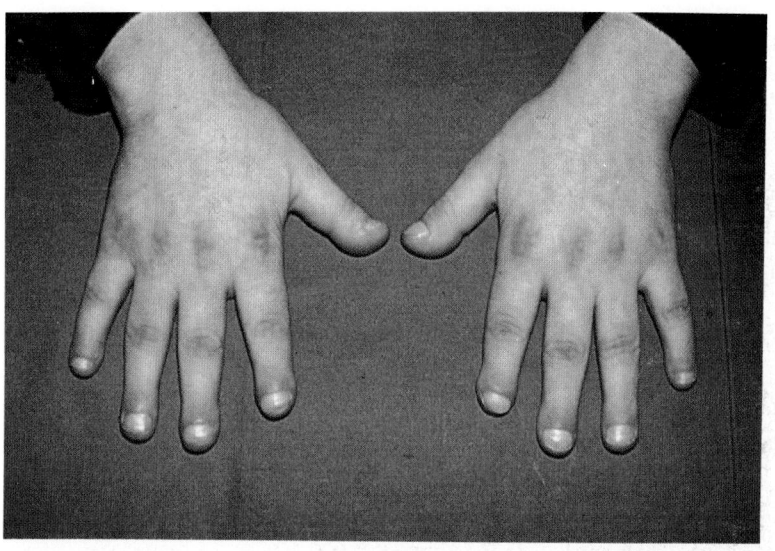

Q 1.20   (a) What is the abnormal physical sign?

(b) What is the diagnosis?

A 1.1   (a) (i) Arthritis of proximal interphalangeal and metacarpal phalangeal joints;

(ii) vasculitis;

(iii) nodule over proximal interphalangeal joint of middle finger.

(b) Rheumatoid arthritis.

Ten to twenty per cent of patients with rheumatoid arthritis form subcutaneous or periostial nodules over pressure points. Such patients may develop vasculitis and are almost invariably seropositive for rheumatoid factors. They tend to develop chronic disease with features of vasculitis, such as neuropathy, chronic skin ulcers, and digital gangrene, and disseminated granulomata affecting the heart, lung, sclera, and dura mater.

A 1.2   (a) Carcinoid syndrome.

(b) Flushing; wheezing; palpitations; facial oedema; abdominal pain.

The carcinoid syndrome results when 5-hydroxytryptophan and 5-hydroxytryptamine, produced by tumours of chromaffin tissue, enter the systemic circulation. Most of these tumours arise in the embryological midgut and, owing to rapid hepatic degradation of 5-hydroxytryptophan and 5-hydroxytryptamine, the syndrome is seen only in cases where metastases to the liver, or beyond, have occurred, or when the primary is situated outside the splanchnic area.

A feature of carcinoid syndrome is facial flushing, which is initially paroxysmal, but eventually leads to cutaneous changes such as multiple fine telangectasiae and a fixed erythematous purple hue to the skin, as seen in slide 1.2.

A 1.3   (a) Bruising in the flank, due to retroperitoneal haemorrhage.

(b) Acute pancreatitis.

(c) (i) Biliary tract disease;

(ii) alcohol.

In acute pancreatitis collections of blood, digested tissue, and pancreatic secretions may burrow along the tissue spaces retroperitoneally into the lesser sac and flank, giving rise to bruising in the costovertebral angle (Grey–Turner's sign). This sign may be seen in any patient who has had a retroperitoneal haemorrhage, causes of which include trauma, bleeding diathesis, and leaking aortic aneurysm. Biliary tract disease and alcohol abuse account for the majority of known factors implicated in acute pancreatitis. Frequently no cause for acute pancreatitis is found but other known causes include:

(i) Metabolic disturbances, including hypercalcaemia, hyperlipidaemia, and diabetic ketoacidosis.

(ii) Infection, e.g. mumps and infectious mononucleosis.

(iii) Trauma, including surgery, endoscopic pancreatography, and pancreatic biopsy.

(iv) Vascular and auto-immune mechanism, e.g. polyarteritis nodosa and systemic lupus erythematosus.

(v) Drugs, including glucocorticoids, immunosuppressive agents, opiates, and oral contraceptives.

Hypothermia.

A 1.4   (a) Dapsone.

(b) Immunofluorescence of the basement membrane may reveal antibody IgA accumulations. Complement and IgA may both be present in normal skin adjacent to active lesions.

Dermatitis herpetiformis is a chronic, intensely pruritic disease of unknown aetiology, which particularly affects males who are middle-aged or older, and may be associated with coeliac disease. The lesions are usually small vesicles with tough walls, although papules and macules occur as well. As the lesions pigment on healing, the affected area may demonstrate active lesions, excoriations, and pigmentation at the same time. The distribution is characteristically symmetrical, the lesions being grouped and concentrated in the interscapular areas of the back, buttocks, the extensor aspect of the forearms, and the scalp. Microscopy of active areas will show vesicles forming at the dermo-epidermal junction. Large numbers of eosinophils occur in the cellular infiltrate, both in the lesions and in the dermis. The immunofluorescent findings mentioned above may be patchy but the skin biopsy should always be examined with this method.

A 1.5   Porphyria cutanea tarda.

Porphyria cutanea tarda is the most common of the hepatic porphyrias. Skin manifestations include a photosensitive dermatitis with hyperpigmentation, a tendency to easy abrasion, skin atrophy, and excessive facial hair growth. Similar cutaneous signs may occur in variegate porphyria, erythropoietic protoporphyria, and congenital erythropoietic porphyria, but not in acute intermittent porphyria.

A 1.6   (a) Dermatomyositis.

      (b) (i) Creatine phosphokinase;

          (ii) electromyography;

          (iii) muscle biopsy.

The rash of dermatomyositis usually consists of an erythema over the face, shoulders, and arms. Erythematous, slightly raised lesions, which sometimes become scaly and atrophic, occur over bony prominences, especially elbows, knuckles, and knees. In childhood, and occasionally in adults, a violaceous suffusion of the upper eyelids, called a heliotrope rash, is diagnostic of dermatomyositis.

Enzymes which derive from muscle are usually elevated in serum. Creatine phosphokinase and aldolase are the most specific, but lactic dehydrogenase and aspartate transaminase are usually elevated also. Electromyography may reveal excessive irritability and polyphasic discharges, the motor units often showing loss of amplitude and shortened duration. Positive denervation waves and fibrillary potentials may be seen, indicating some denervation. Muscle biopsy may reveal inflammatory cells around vessels, which, in the childhood form, may be intense with active arteritis and phlebitis. Individual necrotic muscle fibres are frequently seen in various stages of phagocytosis, along with attempts at regeneration in other fibres.

A 1.7   (a) Diffuse miliary calcification.

      (b) Chickenpox pneumonia.

Pneumonitis due to varicella zoster may complicate chickenpox in about one-third of cases in adults. Respiratory symptoms begin 2–5 days after the eruption. Chest X-rays show diffuse nodular infiltration which may eventually leave a residuum of miliary calcification (Fig. 1A). The differential diagnosis of a similar chest X-ray would include histoplasmosis, haemosiderosis, and tuberculosis.

A 1.8   (i) Brown arc of chronic renal failure;

      (ii) nodule of metastatic calcification in distal phalanx of index finger.

The brown arc, seen in the distal part of the nails, and skin pigmentation are common in slowly progressive renal failure, probably due to melanin and urochromes.

Metastatic calcification is most likely to occur when the serum calcium and phosphate product is high and may involve arteries, periarticular tissue, skin, and eyes.

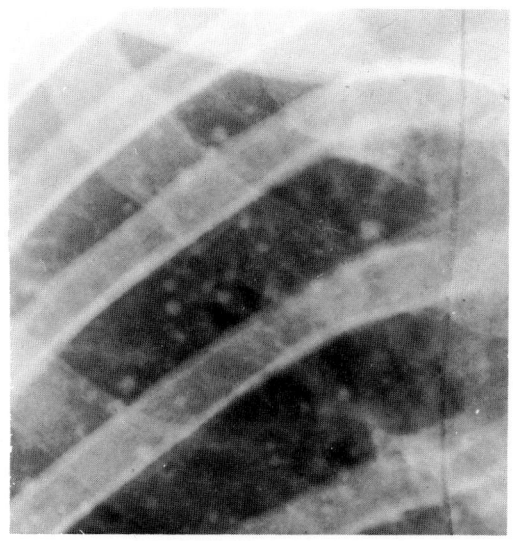

Fig. 1A
A close-up view of the
miliary calcification
following chickenpox
lung infection.

A 1.9   Toxoplasmosis, causing chronic choroido-retinitis.

An area of active choroidal inflammation will show as an ill-defined whitish
opacity, the area being white because it is thicker, thus impairing the normal
red reflex. Exudates of various shades of white, grey, or yellow with arteries
superficial to them characterize choroiditis. If the lesions are chronic the exudates will be surrounded by pigment. Disseminated choroido-retinitis suggests
syphilis. Other causes of choroiditis include tuberculosis and sarcoidosis.

A 1.10   (a) Scleroderma with sicca syndrome.

(b) Schirmer's test for tear production.

The sicca syndrome consists of keratoconjunctivitis sicca and xerostomia. It is
most commonly associated with rheumatoid arthritis, as described by Sjögren,
and to a lesser extent with systemic lupus erythematosus, scleroderma, and
polymyositis, but may also occur in isolation. The sicca syndrome is seen in
10–15 per cent of patients with rheumatoid arthritis, commonly in female
patients with long-standing chronic arthritis.

A 1.11   (a) (i) Exophthalmos;

(ii) thyroid acropachy.

(b) Long-acting thyroid stimulator (LATS).

Pretibial myxoedema, thyroid acropachy, and exophthalmos form a triad of signs found in auto-immune thyroid disease.

Pretibial myxoedema presents as a firm bulging over the antero-lateral aspect of the lower leg. The skin is usually shiny and has an orange-peel appearance. Occasionally similar deposits can be found on the abdomen, hands, or face. Although usually observed at the outset of hyperthyroidism it may occur without associated hyperthyroidism or when the thyroid has been destroyed by thyroiditis. Extremely high levels of LATS are characteristically associated with pretibial myxoedema although no aetiological relationship has been demonstrated.

A 1.12   (a) Xanthelesma.

(b) Primary biliary cirrhosis (PBC).

Ninety per cent of patients with PBC are female, usually aged between 40 and 60 years, who present most frequently with pruritis, with or without jaundice. Secondary hyperlipidaemia may lead to the appearance of xanthelesma, as it may in nephrotic syndrome, diabetes mellitus, and myxoedema.

Immunological abnormalities are common. Ninety-five per cent of cases have circulatory mitochondrial antibodies, an abnormality rarely found in other forms of liver disease. Less specific findings are an elevated serum level of IgM in 80 per cent and circulatory antibodies to the cytoplasm of bile-duct epithelial cells in approximately 75 per cent of cases.

A 1.13   (a) Ruptured Baker's cyst.

(b) Calf pain simulating thrombophlebitis.

Extension of a knee synovial cyst down to the gastrocnemius is usually associated with arthritis and effusion, rheumatoid arthritis being the most common disease predisposing to these cysts. Baker's cysts may rupture and cause calf pain similar to that of deep venous thrombosis or rupture of the gastrocnemic muscle (Fig. 1B).

A 1.14   (a) Handling animal hides or other products contaminated with anthrax spores.

(b) Penicillin or tetracyclines.

Anthrax is now seen almost exclusively in people handling contaminated animal hides or other animal products. The skin lesion usually begins as a small erythematous papule which becomes vesicular and then necrotic, de-

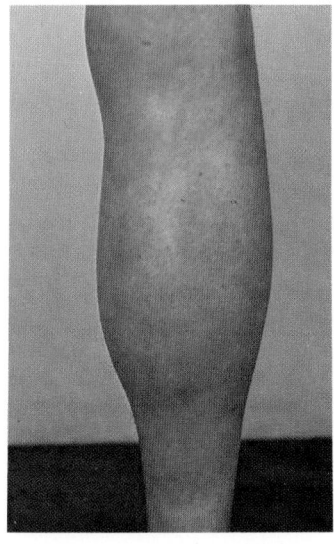

Fig. 1B
Baker's cyst.

veloping a dark crust. Non-pitting oedema often surrounds the eschar and
may extend a considerable distance from it. The lesion is usually pruritic but
not tender and usually occurs on exposed areas. There may be mild regional
lymph node enlargement but lymphangitis may not be observed. Consti-
tutional symptoms and fever are frequently absent, unless the skin disease is
severe or the infection becomes disseminated. Then high fever, prostration,
and death may occur, sometimes with haemorrhagic mediastinitis and
haemorrhagic meningitis.

A 1.15 (a) Asbestosis.

(b) (i) Respiratory failure;

(ii) neoplasia.

Inhalation of asbestos fibres may affect the lungs, leading to pulmonary
fibrosis, and the pleura, giving rise to dense fibrous adhesive pleurisy, plaques,
and calcification (often holly-leaf in configuration). These patients have an
increased risk of developing bronchogenic carcinoma and mesothelioma,
usually of the pleura but occasionally of the peritoneum.

A 1.16 (a) (i) Iron deficiency due to menorrhagia;

(ii) Pernicious anaemia;

(iii) Normocytic or macrocytic anaemia due to hypothyroidism.

(b) Slow rate, low voltage, widespread T-wave flattening.

In myxoedema the skin is thick and dry, with generalized puffiness of the face and extremities. The hair is brittle, straight, and coarse, and eyebrows sparse. The tongue is thick and papillae may be atrophic. Most patients have anaemia. Irregular menstruation and severe menorrhagia frequently occur in younger women with myxoedema. Pernicious anaemia occurs in about one-eighth of patients with idiopathic thyroid failure. Normocytic or macrocytic anaemia may also occur and be related solely to hypothyroidism.

A 1.17 (a) Microangiopathic haemolytic anaemia (MAHA) with (i) frag-mented cells and (ii) burr cells.

(b) (i) Septicaemias, especially gram negative or meningococcal;

(ii) acute progressive malignant hypertension;

(iii) obstetric disorders—antepartum haemorrhage, eclampsia, or post-partum haemorrhage;

(iv) haemolytic–uraemic syndrome.

Additional causes of MAHA include cardiac valve prostheses and patch grafts, exertional haemoglobinuria, thrombotic thrombocytopaenic purpura, and carcinomatosis.

Widespread or localized intravascular deposition of fibrin and platelets damages red cells. In addition to marked fragmentation of red cells with burr cells, helmet cells, microspherocytes, and schistocytes, a peripheral blood film may also show reticulocytosis and moderate to severe thrombo-cytopaenia.

A 1.18 (a) (i) Deforming arthritis;

(ii) dystrophic nails;

(iii) rash.

(b) Arthritis mutilans.

Psoriasis is the most important single cause of deformities of the fingernails. The nail pits are usually small and scattered irregularly over the nail plate. Areas become opaque and patchy discoloration occurs. Subungual hyper-keratosis and onycholysis of the distal edge of the nail plate may also be seen. Nail changes may occur in the absence of skin changes.

Five per cent of patients with skin psoriasis have chronic arthritis.

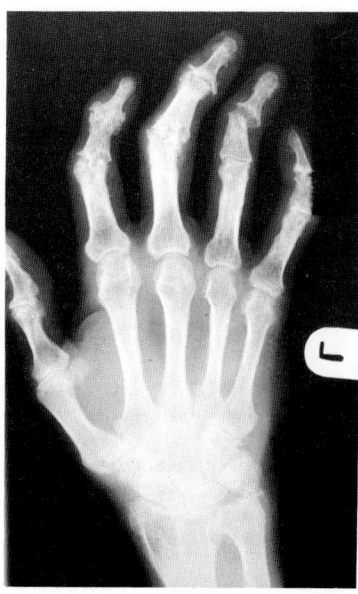

Fig. 1C
This picture of severe osteolytic involvement with resorption of bone and telescoping of digits is characteristic of arthritis mutilans.

Asymmetrical involvement of interphalangeal joints of hands and feet may occur, as may exclusive involvement of distal interphalangeal joints, or a seronegative arthritis, indistinguishable from rheumatoid arthritis. Arthritis mutilans is uncommon and characterized by severe osteolytic involvement with resorption of bone and telescoping of digits (Fig. 1C). Nail involvement is found in about 30 per cent of patients with uncomplicated psoriasis, but rises to over 80 per cent in those with arthritis.

A 1.19   (i) Small left kidney;
             (ii) small dense calyceal volume;
             (iii) delayed early nephrogram.

In the investigation of hypertension an IVP examination must include films during the first few minutes after injection of contrast medium if the delayed early nephrogram of renal artery stenosis is to be seen. Fig. 1D (overleaf) illustrates a smoothly contracted left kidney with a dense pyelogram and smaller calyceal volume than the right kidney, suggesting the presence of left renal artery stenosis. Arteriography is required to demonstrate the anatomical site of the lesion, which may be the result of fibro-muscular hyperplasia (seen more commonly in young patients) or of atheroma (seen more commonly in middle-aged or elderly patients).

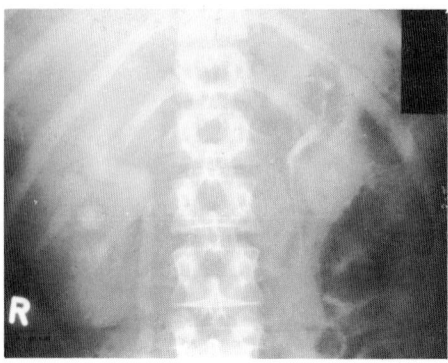

Fig. 1D
An IVP with radiological signs
suggestive of left renal artery
stenosis.

A 1.20   (a) Pseudoclubbing.

(b) Hyperparathyroidism.

Hyperparathyroidism may cause gross resorption of the tufts of the terminal
phalanges, shortening them and giving an appearance similar to clubbing.
However, curvature of the nails in two planes and filling in of the nail angle,
as occurs in clubbing, is not present. The bone disease of hyperparathyroidism
may be recognized radiologically. There may be bone resorption with general
loss of mineral, thinning of the cortices, subperiosteal resorption along the
cortical surfaces of the proximal and distal phalanges, and resorption of the
distal phalangeal tufts (Fig. 1E).

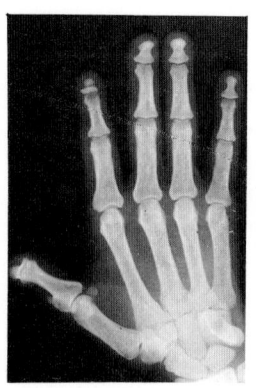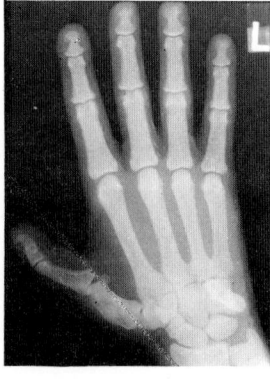

Fig. 1E
Radiograph of the
hands in chronic renal
failure showing gross
resorption of the distal
phalanges and sub-
periosteal erosions.

PAPER 2

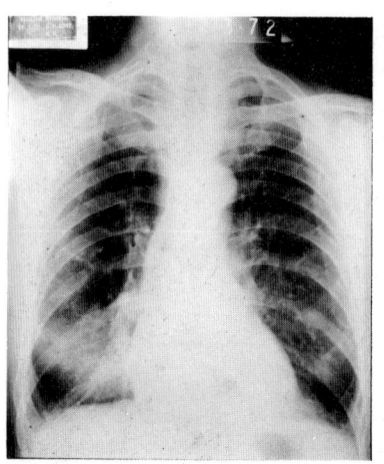 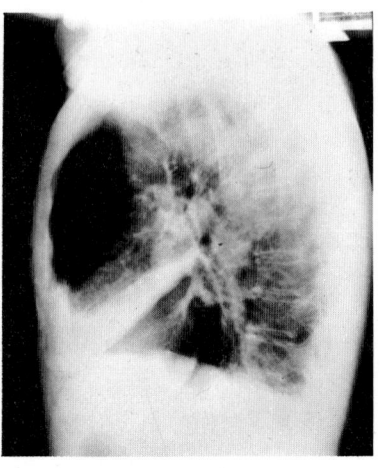

Q 2.1   What is the abnormal radiological sign?

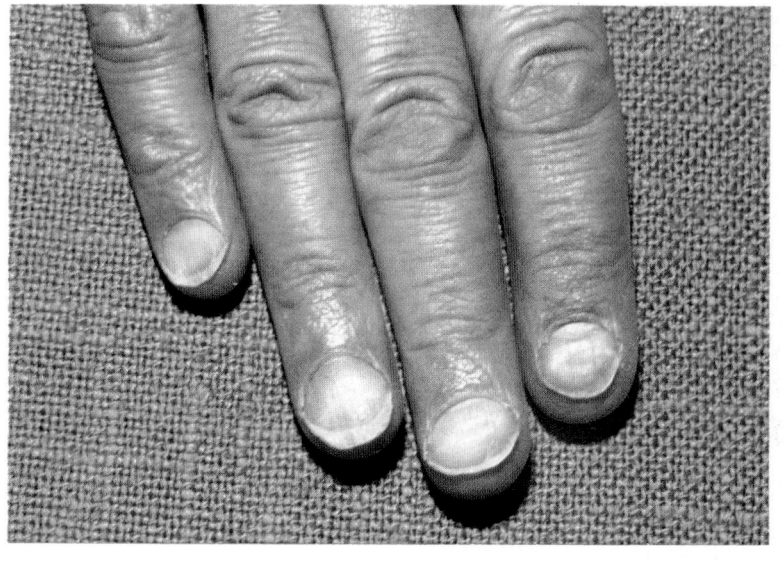

Q 2.2   (a) Name the abnormal physical sign.

(b) With what disorder is this sign associated?

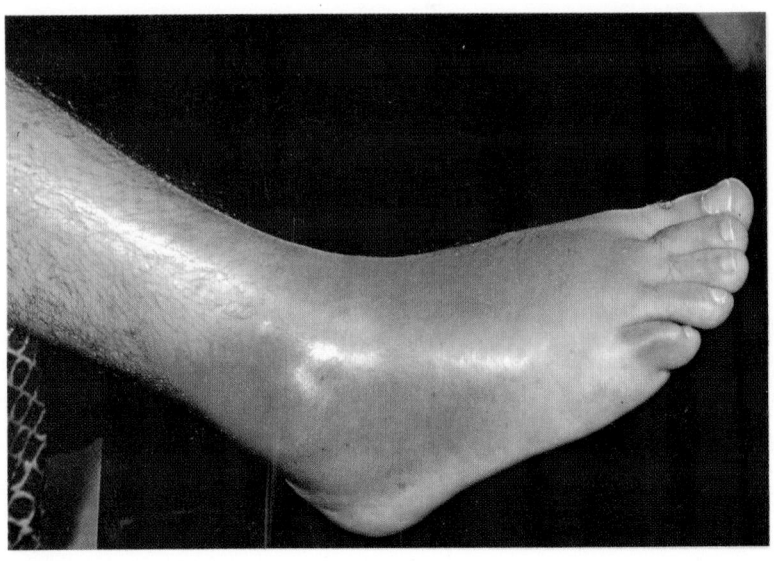

Q 2.3   This patient retired for the night quite well but awakened with excruciating pain in his leg in the middle of the night. The following day thiazide diuretic therapy was stopped.

(a) What is the most likely diagnosis?

(b) What investigation would enable you to make a diagnosis?

(c) Name two other likely causes of a picture like this.

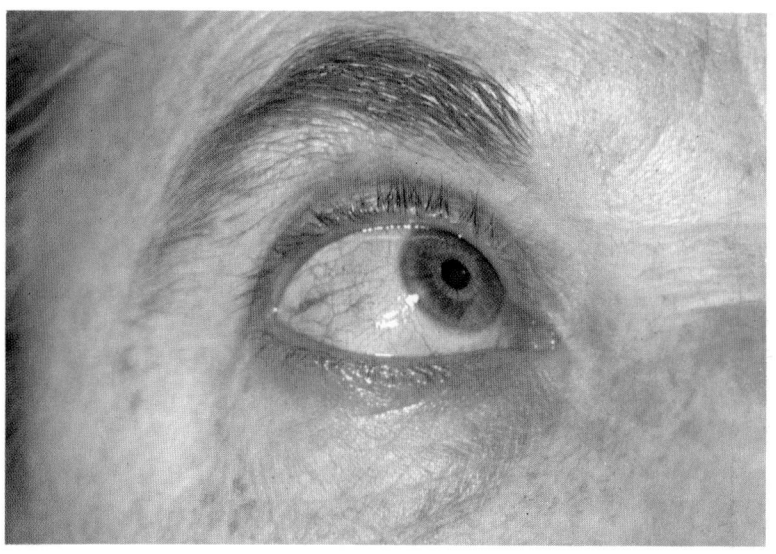

Q 2.4   This patient has suffered several fractures.

(a) What is the abnormal physical sign?

(b) What is the diagnosis?

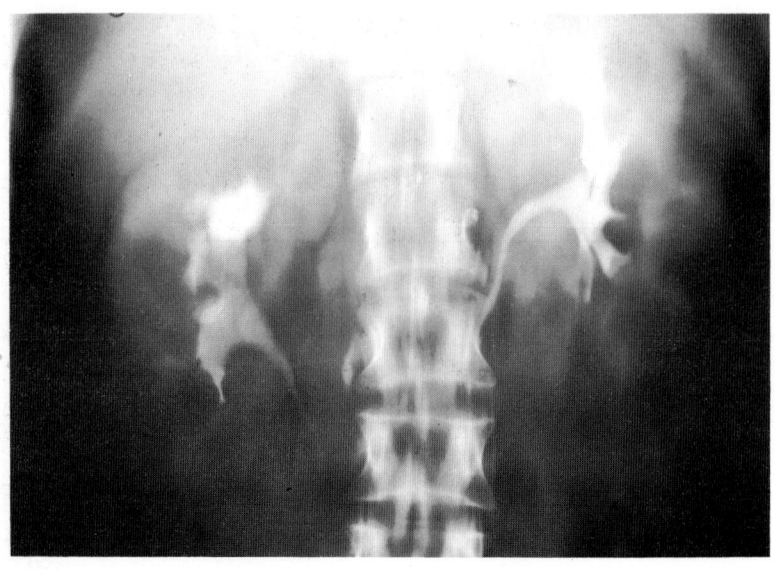

Q 2.5   Give four possible presentations of this disorder.

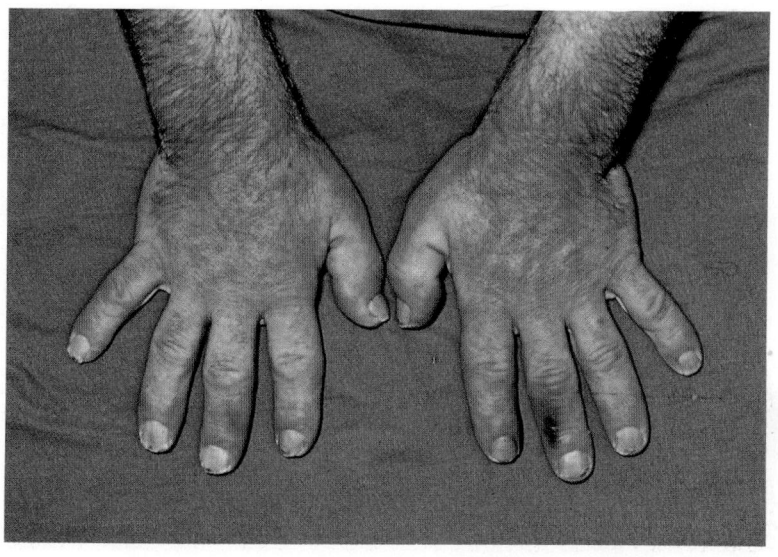

Q 2.6   This patient is impotent.

(a) What is the diagnosis?

(b) Name three investigations you would perform to confirm the diagnosis.

(c) Name the four most common causes of death in this disorder.

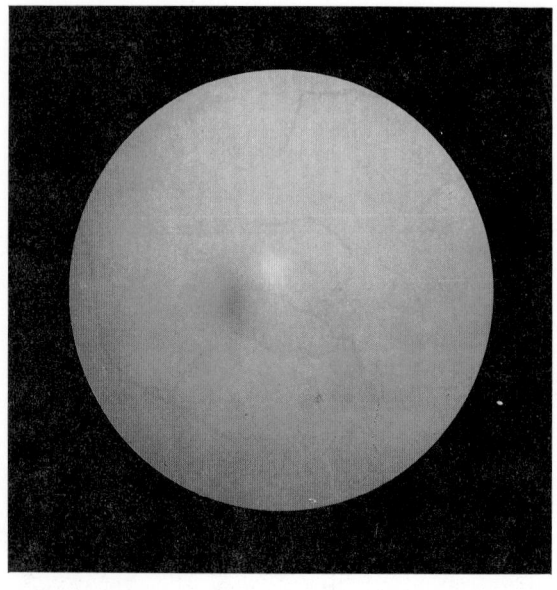

Q 2.7   What is the diagnosis?

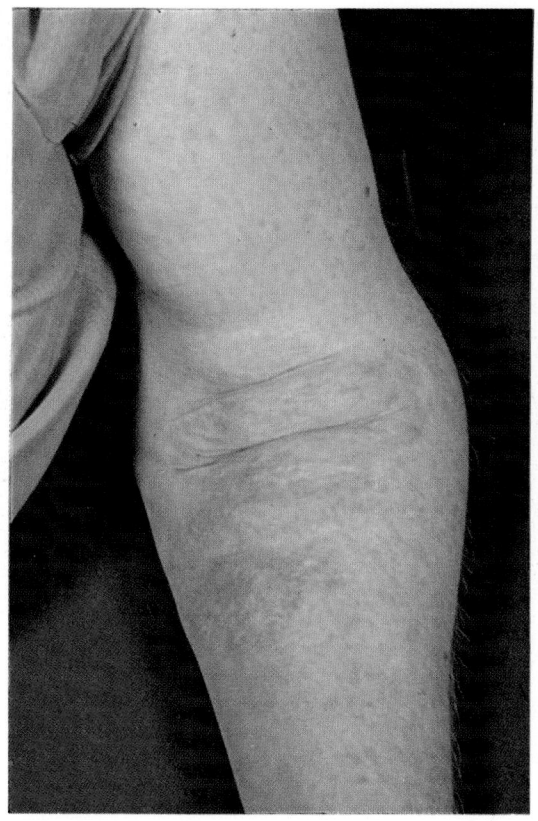

Q 2.8   This 25-year-old patient presented with haematemesis.

      (a) With what disorder are these lesions associated?

      (b) Name two other important complications of this disorder.

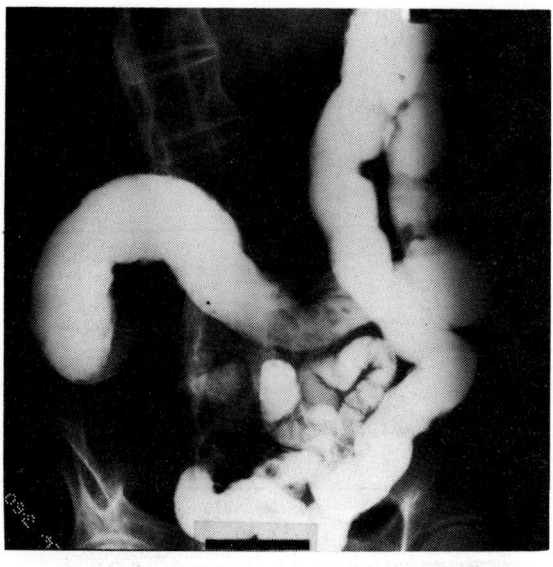

Q 2.9 (a) Radiological evidence of two diseases is present—name both diseases.

(b) Name four life-threatening complications of the colonic disease.

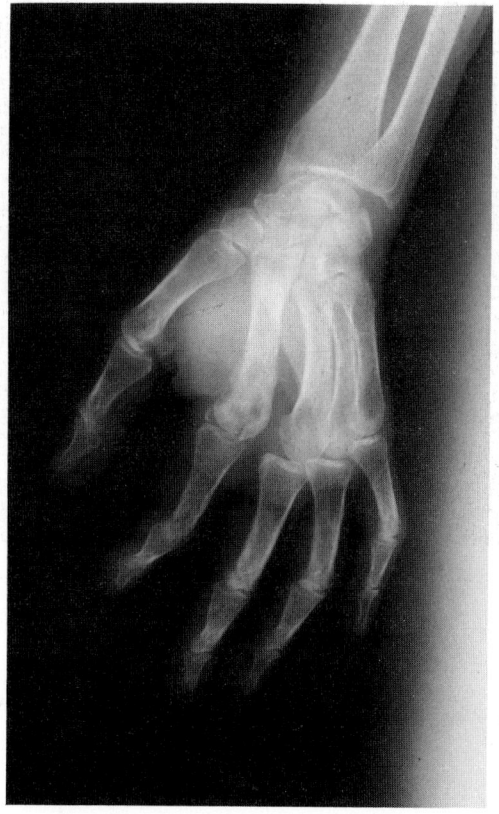

Q 2.10   This Asian man complained of pain and swelling in his hand for one month.

What is the most likely diagnosis?

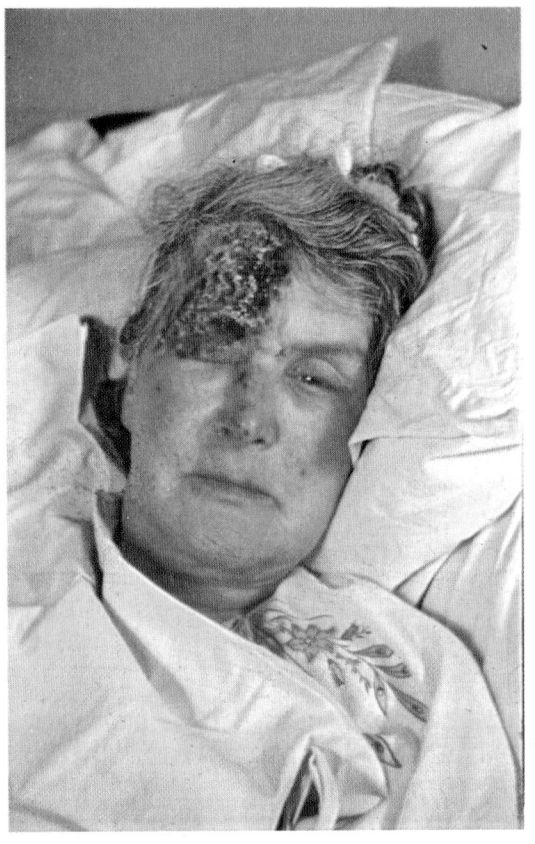

Q 2.11 (a) What is the cause of this lesion?

(b) How would you have treated this problem on appearance of the lesion?

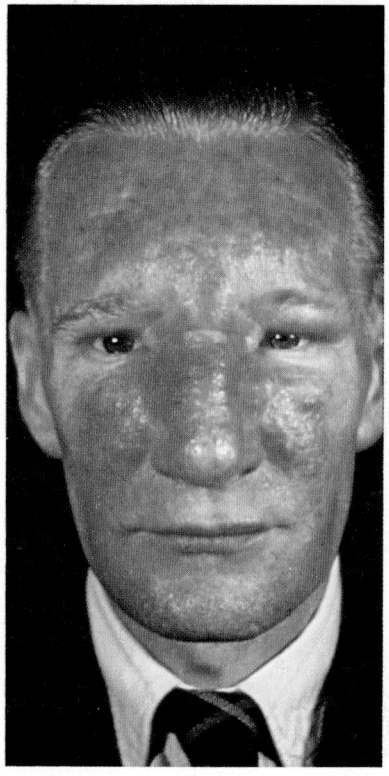

Q 2.12   What is the most serious complication of this disease?

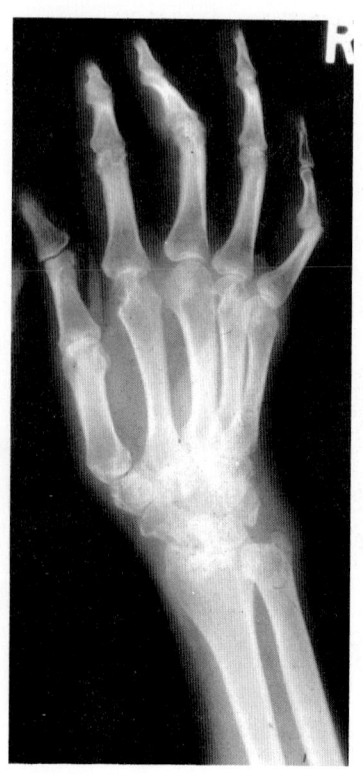 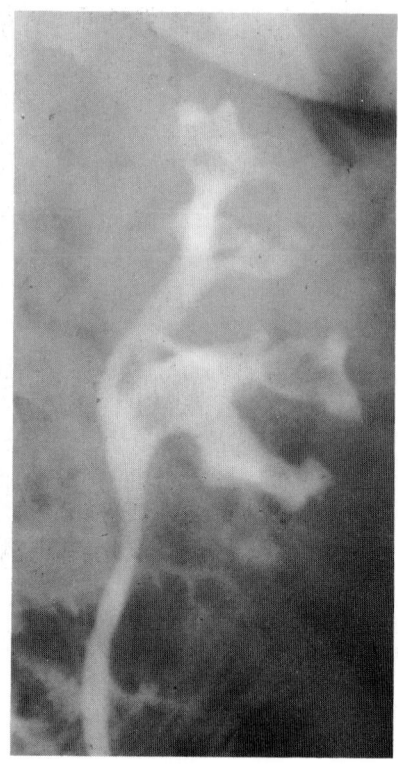

Q 2.13   This patient has had painful hands for several years and presented with colicky abdominal pain.

    (a) What does the hand X-ray illustrate?

    (b) What does the IVP illustrate?

    (c) What is the most likely cause of the renal abnormality in this patient?

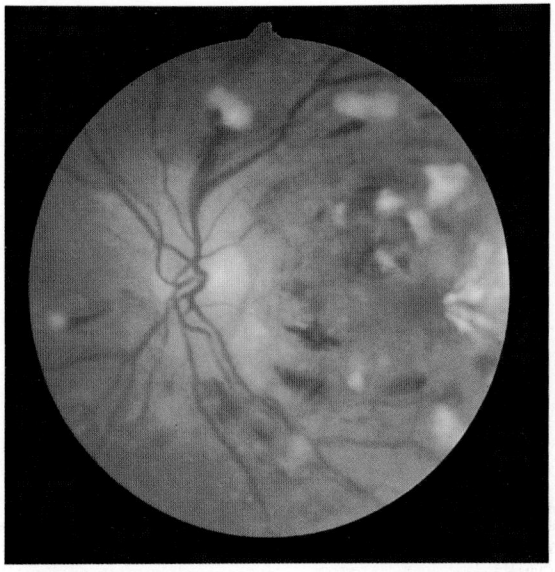

Q 2.14   Name three abnormalities visible in the fundus.

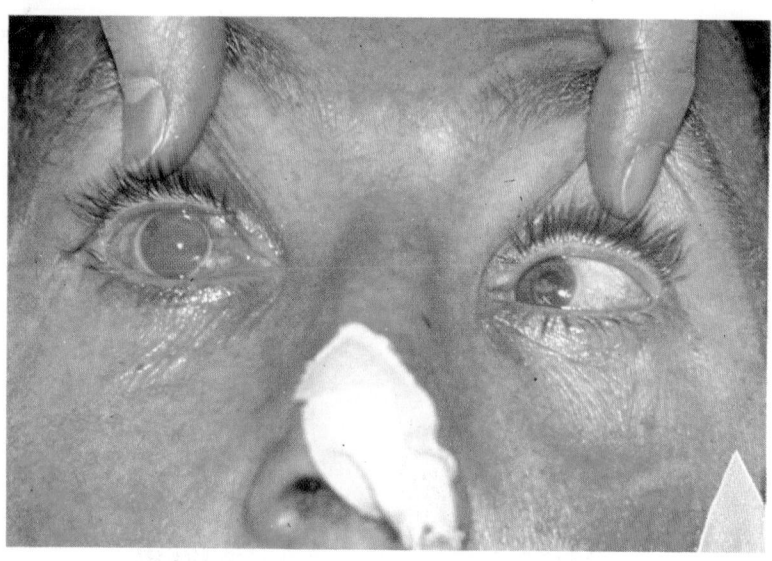

Q 2.15 This patient presented with a painful right eye. Scrotal ulcers were discovered on admission.

(a) Name two abnormal physical signs visible in this patient's eyes.

(b) What is the diagnosis?

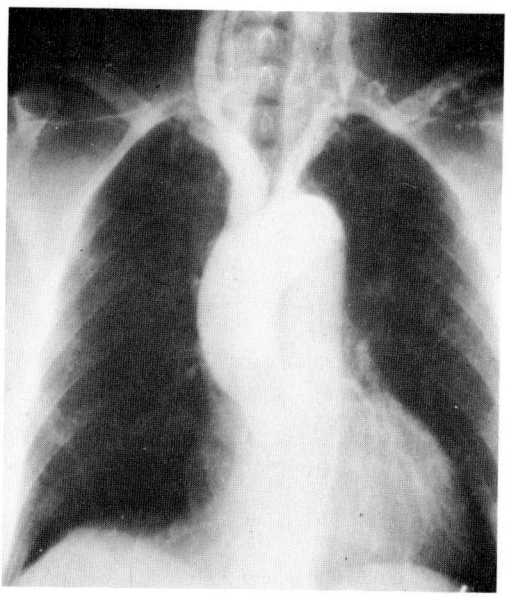

Q 2.16 This young woman presented with fainting attacks and strange feelings in her head, which were attributed to temporal lobe epilepsy.

(a) What abnormalities does the aortogram show?

(b) What is the most likely diagnosis?

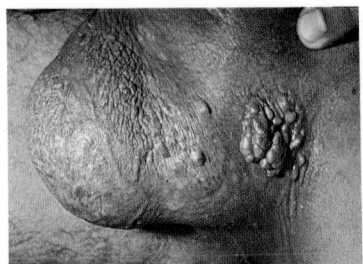
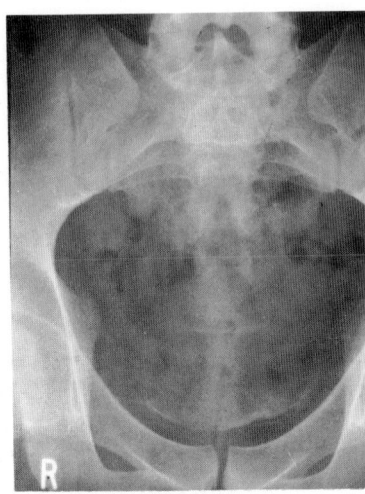

Q 2.17 This patient, from a Middle Eastern country, complained of frequency. In the past he developed an itchy eruption in his groin, similar to the one illustrated, on several occasions after he had gone swimming.

(a) What is the abnormal radiological sign?

(b) What is the cause of the eruption?

(c) How would you make a definitive diagnosis?

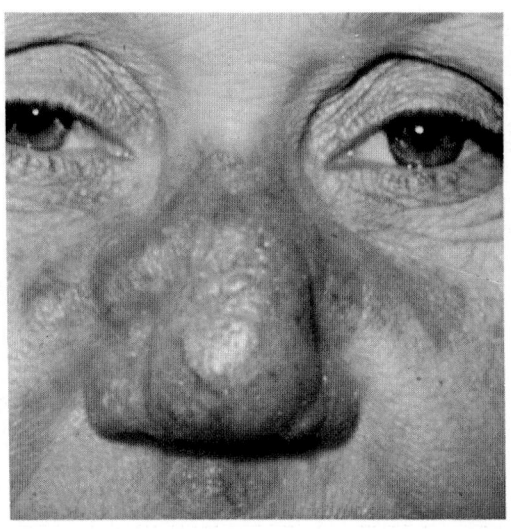

Q 2.18 (a) Name this physical sign.

(b) Name three abnormal physical signs with which this abnormality is frequently associated.

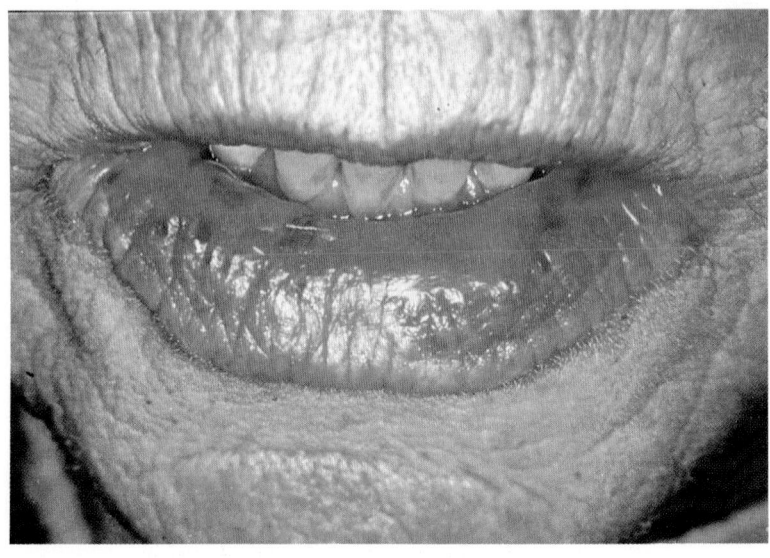

Q 2.19   What is the most important clinical manifestation associated with this physical sign?

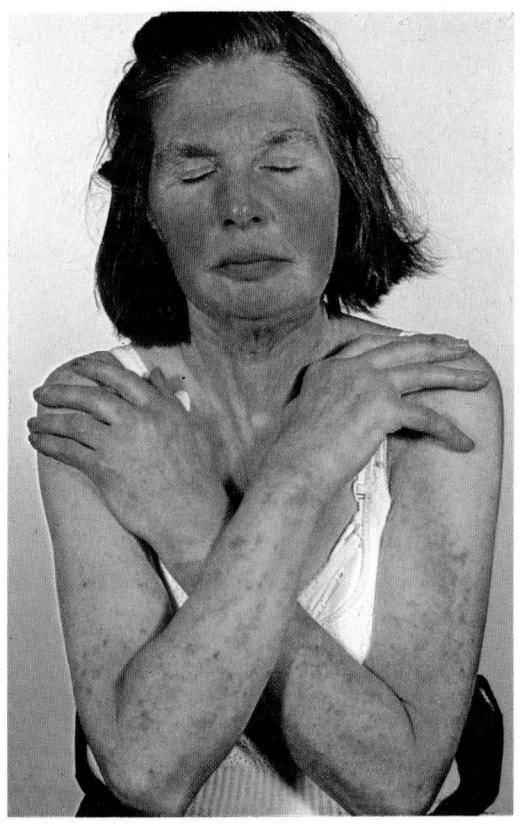

Q 2.20   This patient developed loss of taste within one month of starting treatment.

(a) Name two abnormal signs.

(b) What treatment was commenced?

A 2.1 Right middle lobe collapse and consolidation.

The most important clue to the volume of the middle lobe is provided by the position of the two fissures in the lateral chest X-ray. Usually the lesser fissure can be seen running anteriorly from the hilum to the sternum, with a slight downward bowing. The greater fissure on the right side runs downwards and forwards, from about the level of the fourth or fifth dorsal vertebra, through the hilum, reaching the diaphragm just behind the anterior costophrenic angle. The degree of collapse is indicated by the approximation of the lesser fissure to the lower half of the greater fissure. The increase in radio-opacity is caused by accompanying consolidation. Unless consolidation is marked the postero-anterior projection may show remarkably little evidence of pathology until the collapse is almost complete. Then there is often a loss of clarity of the outline of the right cardiac border.

A 2.2 (a) Koilonychia.

(b) Iron deficiency.

Koilonychia is characterized by loss of the normal convexity of the nail surface which may become flat or concave. The nails lose their normal lustre, becoming thin and brittle. The only important cause of this sign is iron deficiency.

A 2.3 (a) Acute gouty arthritis.

(b) Aspiration of joint fluid for examination with polarized light for needle-shaped birefringent crystals of sodium urate in leucocytes.

(c) (i) Cellulitis;

(ii) septic arthropathy.

The commonest type of acute crystal arthropathy is gout. Acute gouty arthritis may involve one or more joints which rapidly become exquisitely painful. The marked periarticular inflammation may extend to the skin which becomes tense and erythematous. Acute inflammatory changes of heat, marked swelling, extreme tenderness, and rubour extending beyond the joint capsule may raise the possibility of a septic arthropathy or cellulitis. Serum uric acid is usually elevated during an acute attack and intraleucocytic sodium urate crystals are found in over 95 per cent of aspirates from joints affected by acute gout. Rapid response of pain and inflammation to colchicine is characteristic, although indomethacin is the preferred therapy for an acute attack.

A 2.4   (a) Blue sclerae.

(b) Osteogenesis imperfecta.

Osteogenesis imperfecta is an inherited disorder of collagen maturation resulting in defects in connective tissue, which manifest themselves by increased skeletal fragility and blue sclerae. The skin and sclerae are thin. The scleral thinness allows the choroidal pigment to show through, giving a blue tinge, which may also be seen in Marfan's syndrome, and occasionally in patients receiving steroids.

A 2.5   (i) Renal failure;

(ii) haematuria;

(iii) urinary tract infection;

(iv) pain.

There are several types of renal cystic disease, some of which may lead to renal failure.

1. Polycystic disease (PCK)
   (i) Adult PCK disease has a dominant inheritance. It often results in renal failure and is associated with unimportant hepatic and splenic cysts and with Berry aneurysms. This type is by far the most common.
   (ii) Juvenile PCK disease is rare and has an autosomal recessive inheritance. It is associated with hepatic fibrosis.
2. Multicystic disease (renal dysplasia) presents as renal failure or as a renal mass in the neonate and is a consequence of ureteric malformation leading to obstruction *in utero*.
3. Medullary cysts
   (i) Medullary sponge kidney.
   (ii) Medullary cystic disease which causes renal failure in childhood.

In adults a polycystic kidney is usually increased in size and aligned more vertically than normal. Radiographically the calceal systems appear elongated, stretched locally around some cysts, indented locally by others, and occasionally nipped off. The presence of multiple cysts may be confirmed easily by ultrasound.

A 2.6   (a) Acromegaly

(b) (i) Visual field perimetry;

(ii) radiograph of sella turcica;

(iii) radioimmunoassay of plasma growth hormone.

(c) (i) Tumour expansion;

  (ii) cardiac failure;

  (iii) degenerative vascular disease;

  (iv) effects of hypertension.

In acromegaly the hands and feet are enlarged, the increase in subcutaneous connective tissue giving the characteristic thick and fleshy appearance. The extremities may also be hairy with prominent superficial veins. The facial features are blunt and coarse with large ears and nose. The brow is prominent and jaw protruding. The facial wrinkles are exaggerated and the lips full (Fig. 2A).

The course of acromegaly is variable because the onset is usually insidious and because effective treatment may be available. Death may occur within a few years, especially in young people, because of tumour expansion (due to either growth or haemorrhage). In the past, diabetes and hypopituitarism were the usual causes of death, but at present acromegalic heart disease, hypertension, and degenerative vascular disease are the major causes of death in patients with slowly progressive disease.

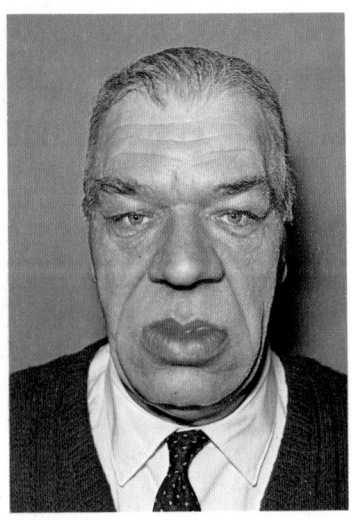

Fig. 2A
The characteristic facies in acromegaly.

A 2.7   Occlusion of central retinal artery.

Occlusion of the central retinal artery causes marked attenuation of the retinal arteries and infarction of the inner layers of the retina, making the retina look pale. The macula lacks the inner layers and receives its blood supply from the choroid. Thus it appears red relative to the surrounding pale

fundus. Death of the nerve cells in the retina leads to degeneration of the optic
nerve and to the development of optic atrophy.

A 2.8   (a) Pseudoxanthoma elasticum.

            (b) (i) Loss of vision;

                 (ii) premature development of atheroma.

Pseudoxanthoma elasticum is a genetically determined disorder of connective
tissue leading to degeneration and calcification of the skin, eyes, and cardiovascular system. Cutaneous lesions are small soft yellowish papules,
arranged parallel to skin lines and folds, and found most often at flexural
areas. Coalescence produces circumscribed or diffuse plaques. In advanced
cases the skin is thick, hangs in loose folds, and resembles the skin of a
plucked chicken.
  Angioid streaks of the retina are the most characteristic eye lesions,
although they may occasionally be seen in patients with Paget's disease or
sickle cell disease. They lie behind the retinal vessels, are most numerous
around the optic discs, and vary in diameter and colour. Premature development of atheroma is common and bleeding from the gastro-intestinal tract
occurs in about 10 per cent of cases.

A 2.9   (a) (i) Ulcerative colitis;

                 (ii) ankylosing spondylitis.

            (b) Toxic megacolon;

                 cancer of the colon;

                 haemorrhage;

                 chronic liver disease.

The radiological changes in acute ulcerative colitis begin with an increase in
mucosal granularity, progressing to visible ulcers which, when extensive, leave
mucosal islands which may look polypoid, and are called 'pseudopolyps'.
Chronic disease leads to a decrease in haustral markings, shortening of the
colon, and narrowing of the lumen. The differential diagnosis between
ulcerative and Crohn's colitis may be difficult, but involvement of the distal
colon in continuity with the rectum and reflux of barium into a dilated,
terminal ileum (backwash ileitis) points to ulcerative colitis.
  The incidence of sacro-ileitis and ankylosing spondylitis in inflammatory
bowel disease is about twenty times that in the general population and, as is
the case with idiopathic ankylosing spondylitis, there is a strong association
with HLA-B27. Sacro-ileitis usually precedes ankylosing spondylitis. The

lateral spinal X-ray in ankylosing spondylitis initially shows filling-in of the concavity of the vertebral bodies, followed by calcification of the anterior and lateral spinal ligaments, with good preservation of the disc spaces. These radiological changes are accompanied by a progressive decrease in spinal mobility and development of the 'bamboo' spine.

A 2.10   Chronic osteomyelitis due to tuberculosis of second metacarpal.

Tuberculosis of bone may induce cystic lytic areas with cortical destruction. Fig. 2B shows the hand swelling which resulted from this patient's bone tuberculosis. Other causes of chronic osteomyelitis include syphilis, gout, and sickle-cell anaemia.

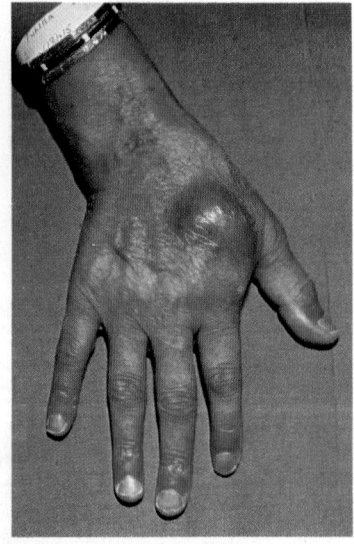

Fig. 2B
A cold abscess due to tuberculous infection of the second metacarpal.

A 2.11   (a) Herpes zoster of the ophthalmic division of the trigeminal nerve, with secondary bacterial infection.

(b) With idoxuridine applied topically.

The lesions are the result of reactivation of the chickenpox virus (varicella zoster) which has lain dormant in the sensory nerves, following an earlier episode of chickenpox. The illness is most likely in those in whom the varicella zoster antibody titre is falling, such as the old and immuno-suppressed.

The lesions are predominantly confined to one or more dermatomes, except in a disseminated infection. The thoracic dermatomes are involved in about

70 per cent of cases and the ophthalmic branch of the trigeminal nerve in about 15 per cent. Pain heralds the appearance of red papules which rapidly vesiculate. Within five to ten days crusting develops which may be confluent.

Treatment comprises idoxuridine applied to the lesions within a few days of appearance of vesicles. In certain cases, where dissemination is judged to be a risk, the systemic anti-viral agent, cytosine arabinoside, is probably of benefit. Hyperimmune globulin may be used as prophylaxis when at-risk subjects have been exposed to varicella zoster virus.

A 2.12　Keratitis, with corneal vascularization and opacity.

Rosacea is most common in middle-aged women. It tends to occur in the easy flusher in whom environmental factors, such as alcohol and sunlight, may induce facial hyperaemia. Progression is accompanied by permanent secondary telangiectasiae. Occasionally rhinophyma occurs in those with a tendency to seborrhoea, especially men. Keratitis may be severe leading to corneal vascularization, and sometimes to blindness.

A 2.13　(a)　Erosive arthropathy of rheumatoid distribution.

　　　　　(b)　Papillary necrosis.

　　　　　(c)　Analgesic nephropathy.

Radiological signs of rheumatoid arthritis include soft tissue swelling, juxta-articular osteoporosis, reduction in joint space, and bony erosions, especially of proximal interphalangeal joints, metacarpo-phalangeal joints, and carpus.

The ingestion of large quantities of phenacetin-containing analgesics may cause an interstitial nephritis, with or without papillary necrosis. It has in the past been a significant cause of renal disease in rheumatoid patients. The role of other analgesics in the genesis of these lesions is much less clear-cut. The radiological changes of papillary necrosis are the result of excavation or sloughing of the papillae and occur late in the disease. A sloughed papilla remaining *in situ* may be surrounded by a ring of contrast. Subsequent displacement of the papilla leaves a defect which makes the calyx appear clubbed, and allows the excavated space to fill with contrast material. Excavations of this type may also occur in diabetes mellitus, sickle-cell disease, and to a lesser extent in chronic alcoholism, tuberculosis, and atrophic pyelonephritis.

A 2.14　Arterial narrowing, arteriovenous crossing changes, hard exudates, macular star.

Replacement fibrosis in the retinal arterioles usually develops in slowly increasing, moderately severe hypertension, associated chiefly with elevation of systolic blood-pressure in the 170–200 mm Hg range, with diastolic blood-pressure around 100 mm Hg. This causes attenuation and tortuosity of arterioles, changes in the vascular light reflex (such as widening, copper and silver wiring, irregularities of calibre), arteriovenous crossing changes, hard shiny exudates, and haemorrhages (usually superficial and minute). As the light reflex broadens it occupies most of the width of the blood vessel and light of poor intensity may give metallic reflections called copper wiring. As replacement fibrosis continues, the vessel wall obscures the blood column and the arteriole appears as a whitish tube containing a red fluid (silver wiring). The hard shiny exudates that develop in areas of chronic retinal ischaemia are lipid-laden macrophages, and occur in the inner layers of the retina.

Fibrinoid necrosis of the arterioles, which usually develops only when the diastolic blood-pressure is extremely high, is part of the clinical picture of 'accelerated hypertension'. Retinal changes include severe attenuation of arterioles, retinal oedema, fluffy cotton-wool exudates, haemorrhages, and papilloedema (Fig. 2C). Haemorrhages may occur in the nerve fibre layer and, following spread in the plane of the fibres, appear linear or flame-shaped. Cotton-wool spots are also located in the nerve fibre layer. They may be caused by arteriolar necrosis or spasm, giving rise to infarction and abnormal endothelial permeability. A macular star consists of foam cells grouped between the radial fibres of the macula producing glistening yellowish-white exudates. Signs of fibrinoid necrosis in the retina imply its presence in other vascular beds, the two most important being in the central nervous system and kidneys, where it may cause hypertensive encephalopathy and renal failure respectively.

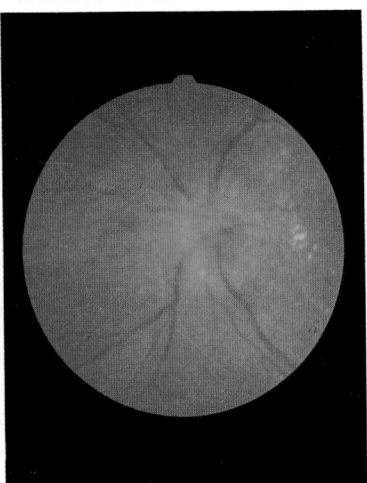

Fig. 2C
This photograph illustrates the papilloedema, cotton-wool exudates, and attenuation of aterioles which occurs in grade 4 hypertensive retinopathy. The grading system is that of Keith–Wegener–Barker, the most widely used grouping of retinal changes associated with hypertension.

A 2.15   (a) (i) Left sixth nerve palsy;

(ii) right iritis.

(b) Behçet's disease.

Behçet's disease is a multi-system disorder with a variety of clinical manifestations, of which oral, genital, ophthalmic, neurological, and musculo-skeletal are the most important.

The genitalia may be affected by pyodermas, herpes-like lesions, or ulcers (Fig. 2D). Eye involvement is the most frequent cause of disability, the most common lesions being iridocyclitis and uveitis, which may be severe and lead to loss of vision. Neurological complications include cranial nerve palsies, meningoencephalitis, psychosis, and, rarely, peripheral neuropathy.

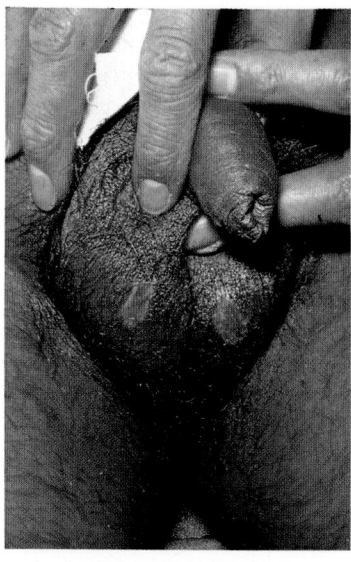

Fig. 2D
Scrotal ulcers in a patient with Behçet's syndrome.

A 2.16   (a) Constrictions of the junction of the subclavian and carotid arteries.

(b) Aortic arch syndrome.

Occlusion of the vessels arising from the arch of the aorta is termed aortic arch syndrome or pulseless disease. Today the majority of patients of middle and older age groups with this disorder have atheroma, whereas in the past syphilitic arteritis was a common cause. Pulseless disease may also be due to obstructive lesions in arteries associated with supravalvar aortic stenosis. A non-specific arteritis called Takayashu's disease is a well-known but rare cause of aortic arch syndrome which occurs most frequently in females and which is usually diagnosed during the third decade of life.

A 2.17 (a) Bladder wall calcification.

(b) Allergic reaction to schistosome cercariae.

(c) Look for schistosome eggs in the urine or in a biopsy of rectum or bladder.

Schistosomiasis begins with penetration of the skin by cercariae which are found in infected fresh water. The organism dies in the skin and its break-down products produce a cutaneous allergic reaction. Subsequent exposures result in immediate urticarial wheals, followed by papules with an erythematous halo, vesicles, and pustules, which subside within a week.

Severe urinary tract schistosomiasis may occur in both early and late phases of infection with *Schistosoma haematobium*. Initially, granulomatous inflammatory rections to the eggs in both the ureter and bladder may cause ureteral obstruction. As the disease progresses irreversible fibrosis with diffuse calcification develops, leading to frequency and dysuria.

Definitive diagnosis can be made only by finding schistosome eggs in the urine or in a biopsy specimen. There is a diurnal variation in egg excretion. Therefore urine should be collected at mid-day, centrifuged, and the sediment microscoped. Rectal biopsy, when examined immediately, is a highly efficient way of diagnosing schistosomiasis including that due to *S. haematobium*. On cystoscopy sandy patches made of schistosome eggs may be seen on the bladder wall.

A 2.18 (a) Lupus pernio.

(b) Chronic sarcoidosis of:

(i) Skin: plaques, scars, keloids;

(ii) eyes: keratoconjunctivitis sicca, chronic uveitis;

(iii) lung: pulmonary fibrosis.

Lupus pernio is one of the cutaneous signs of chronic sarcoidosis which, unlike the acute form, tends to progress inexorably and responds poorly to treatment. Pulmonary fibrosis is the most serious complication, but uveitis and hypercalcaemia may also give rise to serious morbidity in chronic sarcoidosis. Clearing of the abnormal chest X-ray of sarcoid fibrosis occurs in only one-fifth of patients with skin lesions.

Lupus vulgaris is a sign of long-standing cutaneous tuberculosis which may ulcerate and destroy nasal tissue. Small, multiple, amber-coloured plaques or nodules enlarge and form a roughly circular lesion, in which atrophy and scarring occur in the centre. Long-term lesions may be quite disfiguring as a result of scarring. Acid-fast bacilli are present in the lesion. It is more important to recognize tuberculosis than to overlook sarcoidosis, as the former disease will respond quickly to antituberculous drugs.

A 2.19 Gastro-intestinal polyposis.

The Peutz–Jegher syndrome, which is an autosomal dominant inherited condition, comprises gastro-intestinal polyposis and mucocutaneous pigmentation, the latter involving the buccal mucosa, perioral and periorbital skin, and distal extremities. The majority of polyps, which are hamartomas, occur in the jejunum and ileum, but gastric (Fig. 2E) and colorectal polyps may also be present. Rarely the polyps may become malignant.

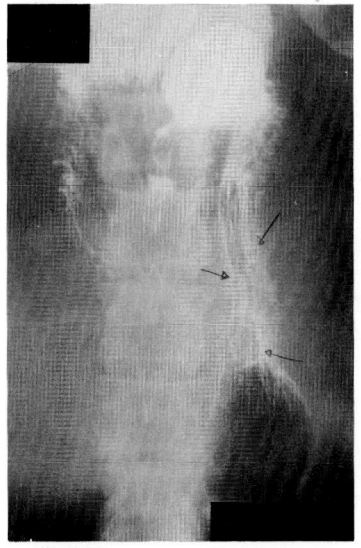

Fig. 2E
Gastric polyps (arrowed) in Peutz–Jegher's syndrome.

A 2.20   (a) (i) Rash on arms and face;

(ii) hand arthritis of rheumatoid distribution.

(b) Pencillamine.

Although rashes, especially with butterfly distribution, may occur in connective tissue disease, drugs are the most likely cause of a rash in rheumatoid arthritis. Gold and penicillamine in particular may induce dermatitis. Penicillamine treatment may precipitate loss of taste, thrombocytopaenia, proteinuria, anorexia, nausea, and vomiting.

PAPER 3

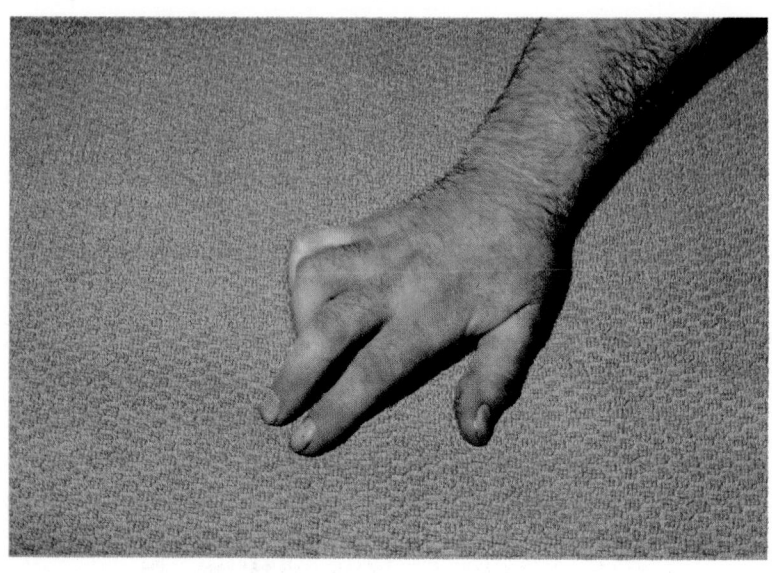

Q 3.1   This patient dislocated his elbow 10 years previously while playing rugby.

Which muscles in the hand are not weak?

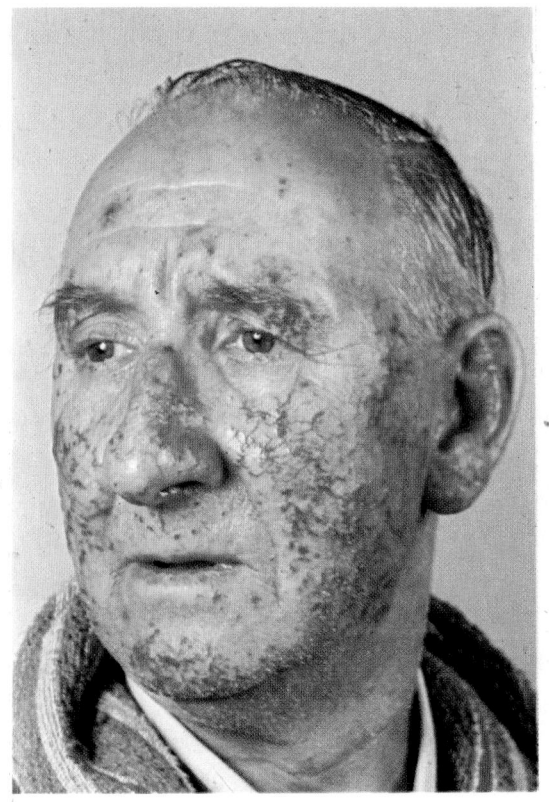

Q 3.2   (a) What is the most likely diagnosis?

(b) What is the most important complication of this disease?

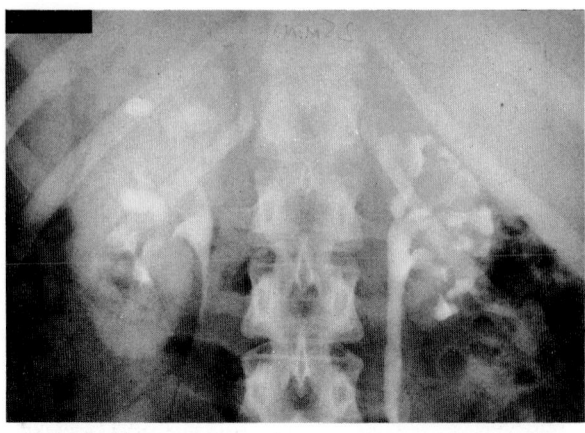

Q 3.3 This 10-year-old girl complained of haematuria for one week. Of what disorder is this IVP characteristic?

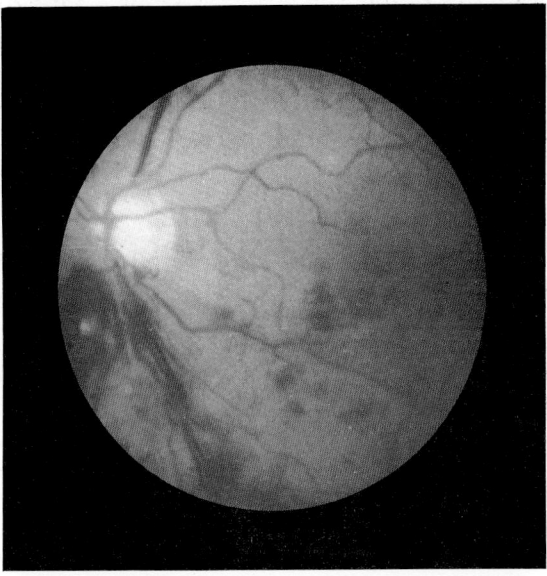

Q 3.4   (a) Name two abnormalities.

(b) What is the diagnosis?

(c) What is the most likely cause of this disorder?

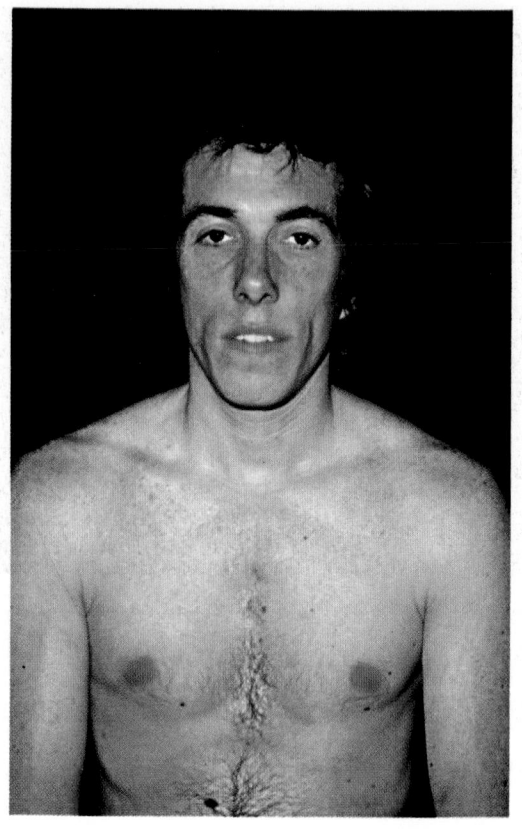

Q 3.5 The patient is in renal failure and has a persistent reduction in serum C3 complement.

(a) Name the abnormal sign.

(b) With what disease is this sign associated?

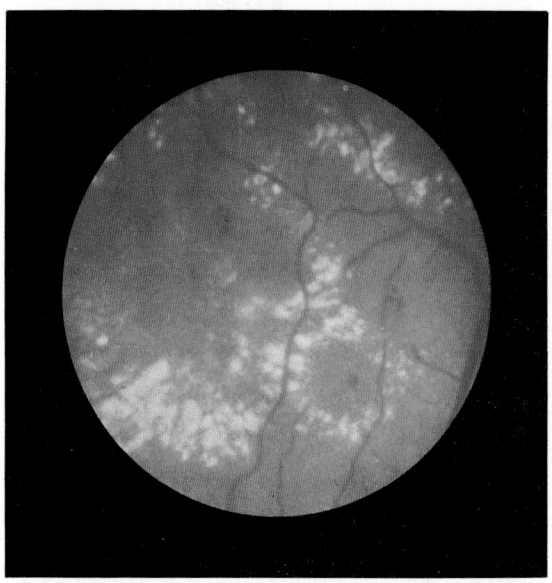

Q 3.6   (a) What is the diagnosis?

(b) Name three other complications from which this patient may suffer.

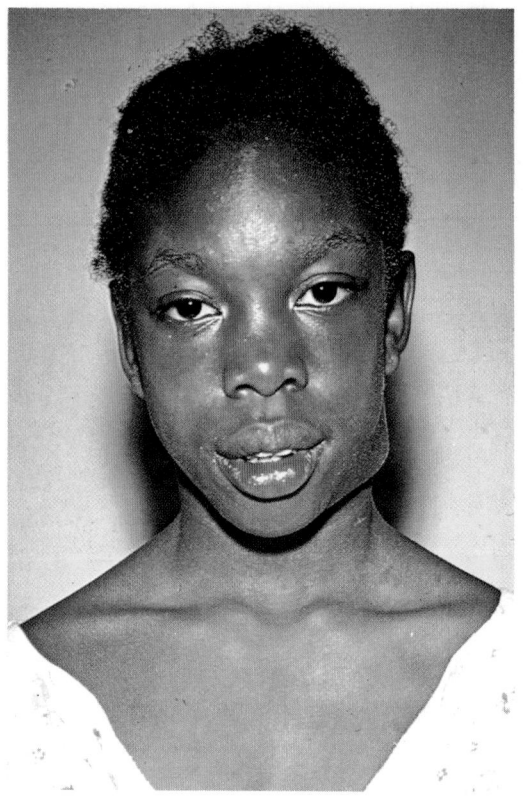

Q 3.7 This patient presented, soon after arriving in England from a West Indian rural community, with anorexia and fatigue of two months' duration.

(a) What is the most likely cause of the lesion visible on the slide?

(b) What single investigation would you do to confirm the diagnosis?

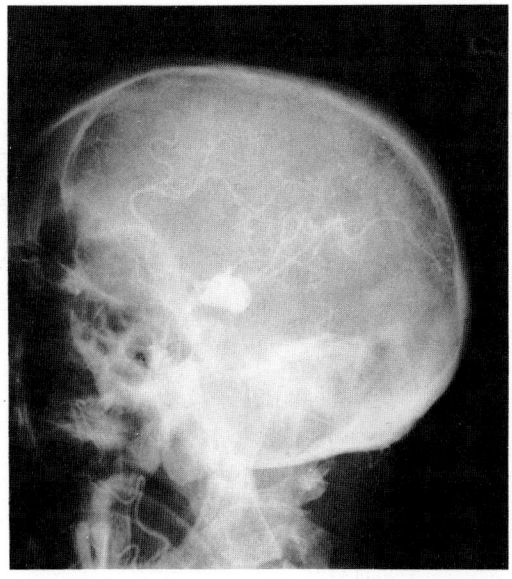

Q 3.8   This patient developed diplopia suddenly.

(a) Where is this abnormality?

(b) Name the two major presentations of this disorder.

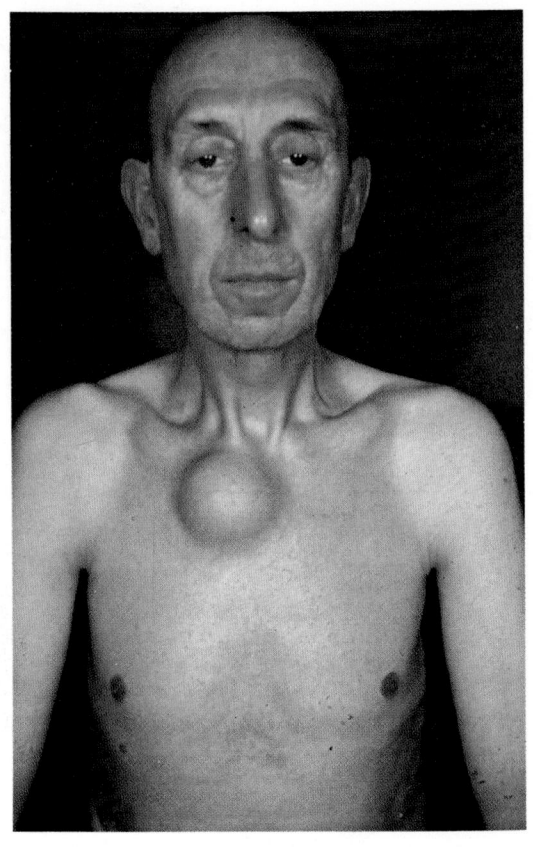

Q 3.9   This patient attended his doctor because he had developed par-
oxysms of coughing. The pulsatile mass was mentioned *en passant*.

(a) What is the cause of this lesion?

(b) What is the most likely cause of this cough?

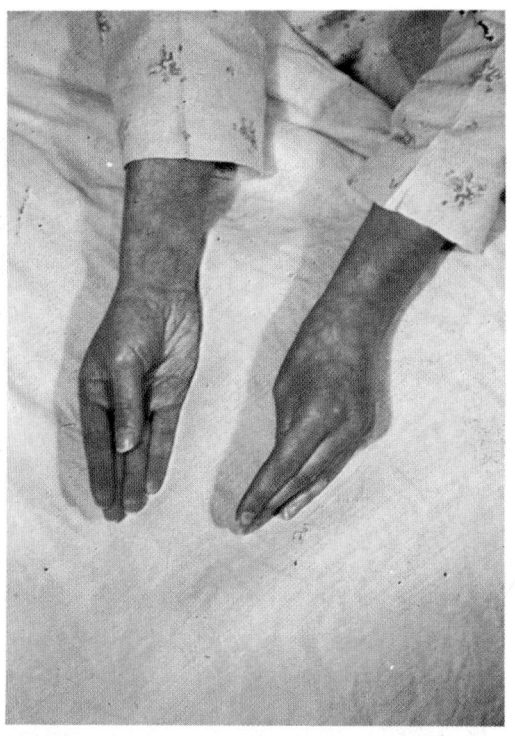

Q 3.10   This patient's gag reflex was absent.

    (a) What is the abnormal physical sign?

    (b) What is the most likely diagnosis?

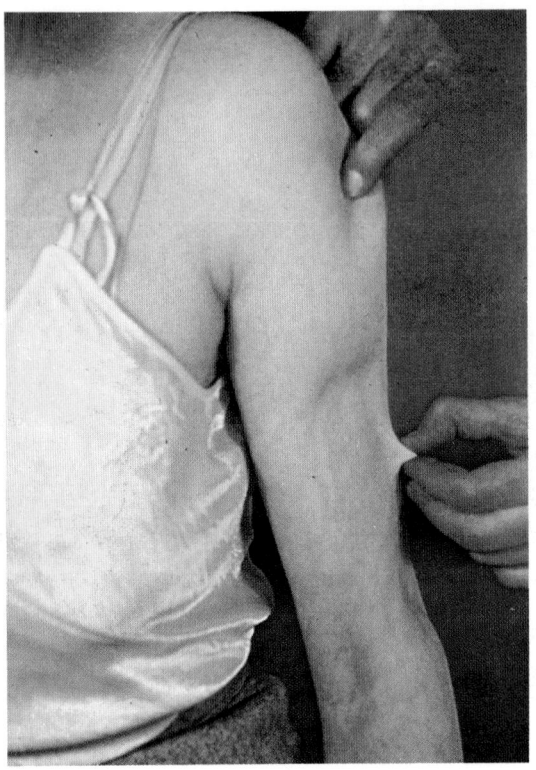

Q 3.11 This lady was brought to the casualty department having been found comatose.

(a) What is the abnormal physical sign?

(b) What immediate investigation would you do?

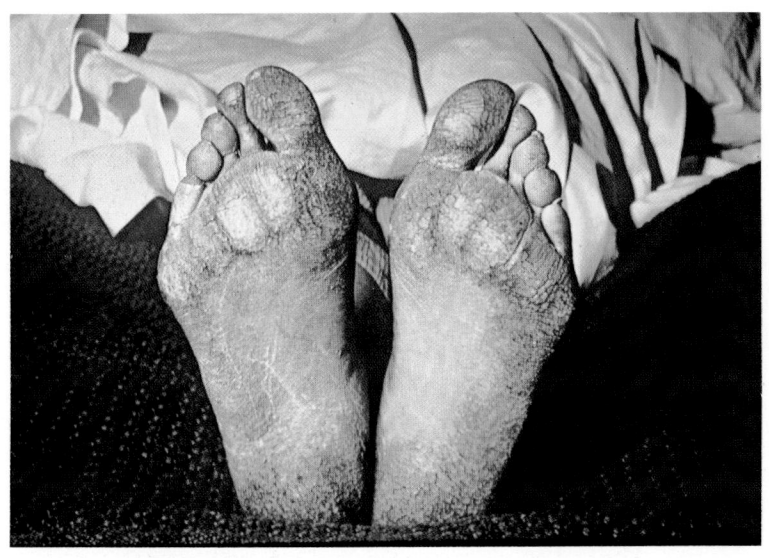

Q 3.12   This patient complains of difficulty in swallowing food.

(a) What is the abnormal physical sign?

(b) What is the cause of the dysphagia?

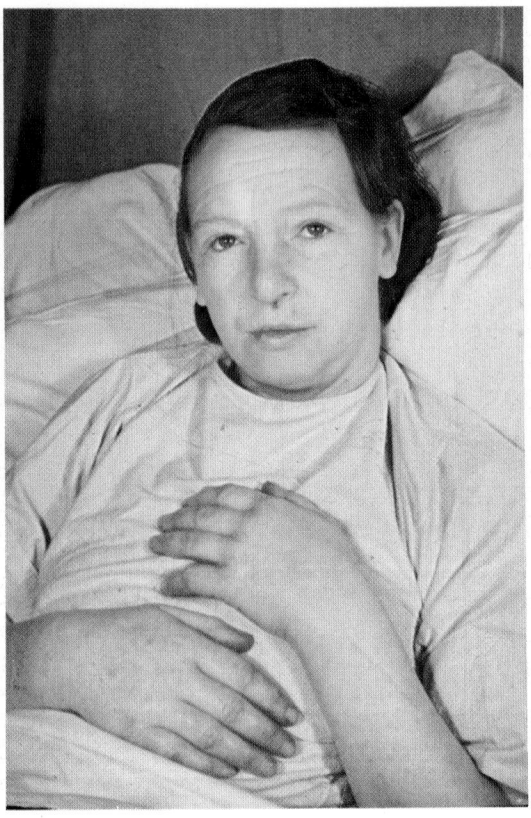

Q 3.13   This 40-year-old lady had been referred to the psychiatric department complaining of weakness and lethargy for the previous year.
Her haemoglobin is normal.

(a) What is the diagnosis?

(b) What are the two most likely causes of this disorder?

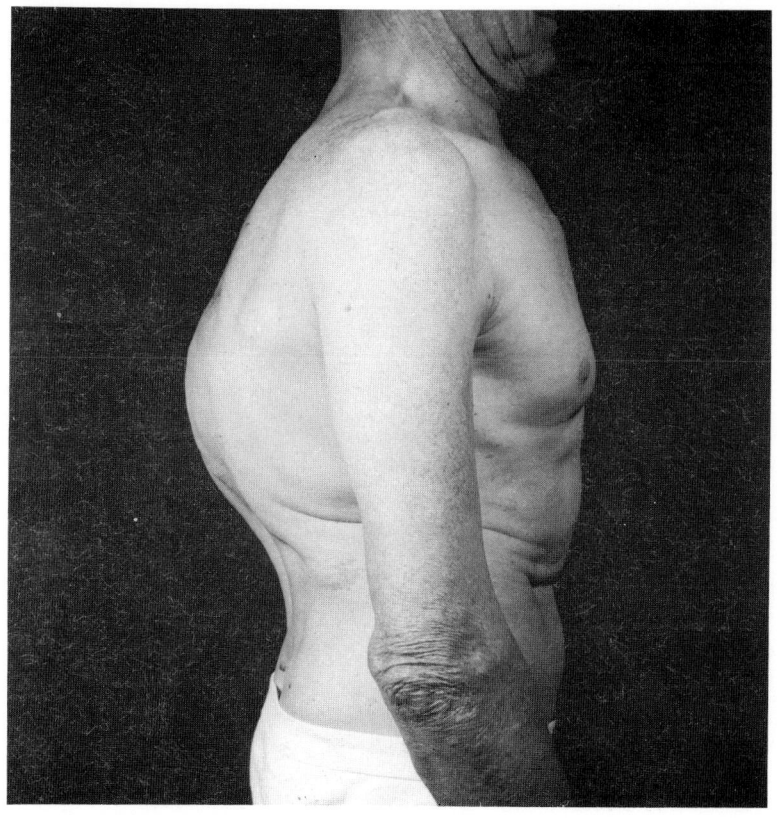

Q 3.14   (a) What is the abnormal physical sign?

(b) What is the most likely diagnosis?

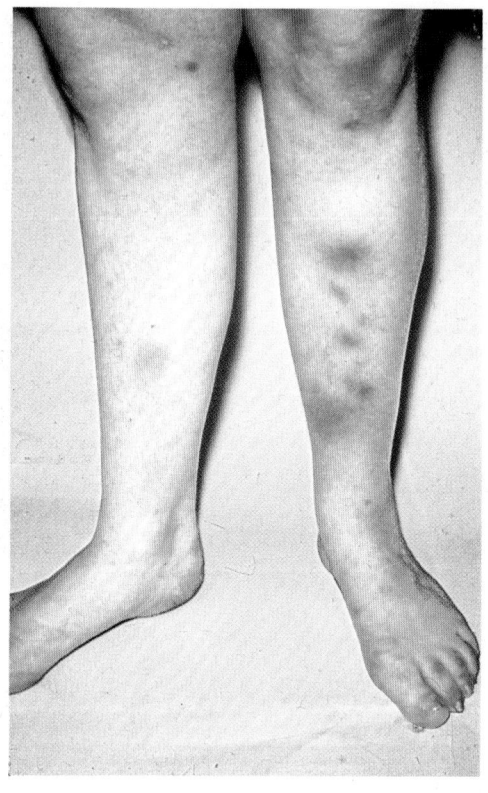

Q 3.15 What are the four most likely causes of this physical sign in Britain?

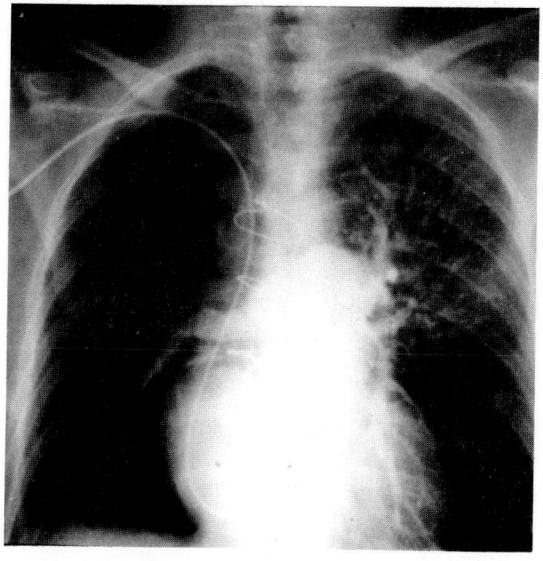

Q 3.16 (a) What is the diagnosis?

(b) Name two ECG patterns which are characteristic of this disorder.

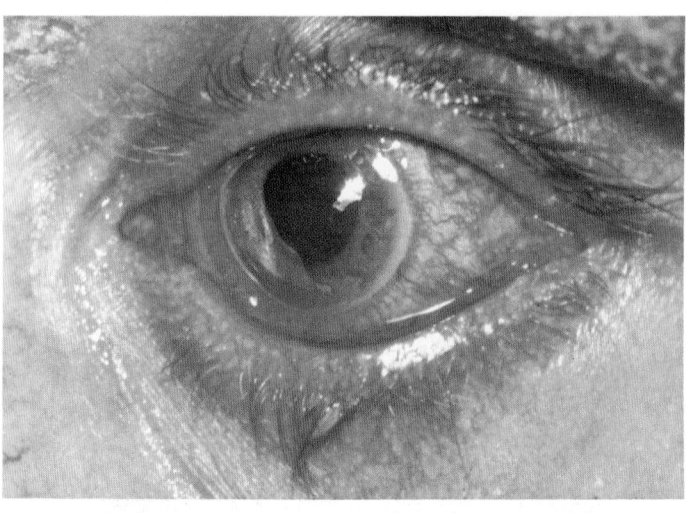

Q 3.17 (a) Name the abnormal physical sign.

(b) Name five generalized diseases associated with this physical sign.

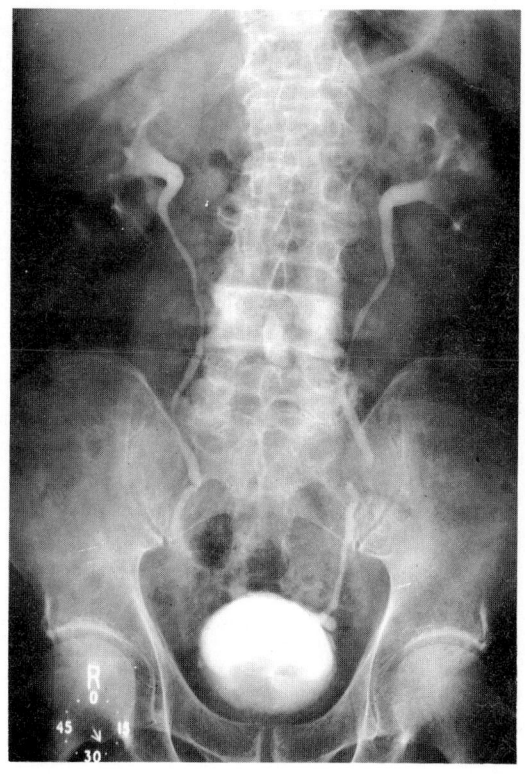

Q 3.18   (a) What is the abnormality visible on this X-ray?

(b) Name the two most likely causes of this picture.

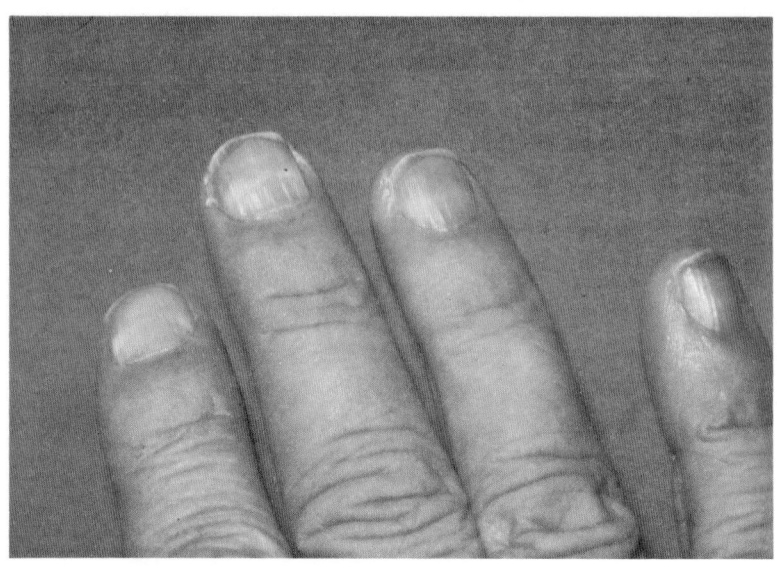

Q 3.19 Name three causes of this physical sign.

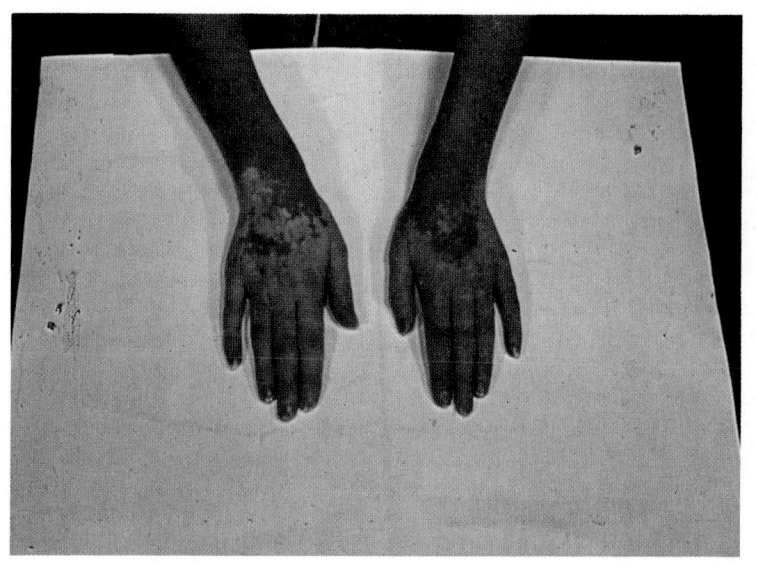

Q 3.20   This patient is Irish.

(a) Name two abnormal clinical signs.

(b) What is the most likely diagnosis?

A 3.1   Lateral two lumbricals; opponens pollicis; abductor pollicis brevis; outer head of flexor pollicis brevis.

Complete ulnar nerve paralysis results in a claw hand deformity due to weakness and wasting of the small hand muscles, hyperextension of the fingers at the metacarpophalangeal joints, and flexion at the interphalangeal joints. The flexion deformity is most pronounced at the ring and little fingers. The ulnar nerve is most commonly damaged at the elbow, following fracture or dislocation. In the hand the ulnar nerve innervates the small muscles, except abductor pollicis brevis, opponens pollicis, the lateral two lumbricals, and the outer head of flexor pollicis brevis, these being innervated by the median nerve. Involvement of all the small muscles of the hand is seen in T_1 root lesions, as well as in combined ulnar and median nerve palsies.

A 3.2   (a) Hereditary haemorrhagic telangiectasiae.

(b) Gastro-intestinal bleeding.

Telangiectases involve arterioles, capillaries, and venules and have very thin vessel walls which balloon. Whether flat or raised, telangiectases blanch with pressure. Similar lesions may occur in scleroderma. In the inherited disorder the lesions are common on the face and in the mucous membranes of the tongue, lips, and nose. Visceral lesions are common, particularly in the gut. Pulmonary arteriovenous fistulae occur in about one-fifth of patients.

A 3.3   Chronic pyelonephritis.

The most frequently occuring disease of the kidneys in British children is chronic focal pyelonephritis. The scars in this disorder are usually large enough to distort the renal outline and the internal pattern of pyramids and calyces. The kidneys are shrunken, and the cortex overlying the scars is thin, the scars becoming more obvious as the healthy tissue grows. When severe disease is present the calycine structures of both kidneys become grossly distorted and there are multiple unequally distributed areas where the renal substance is extremely thin. Focal cortical scarring with preservation of the papillae and normal calyces suggests renal ischaemia rather than chronic pyelonephritis.

A 3.4   (a) Dilated inferior temporal vein with (i) oedema and (ii) haemorrhage in area of drainage.

(b) Occlusion of tributary of central retinal vein.

(c) Atheroma at an arterio-venous crossing.

Arteries and veins are bound together in a common adventitial sheath at the lamina cribrosa at arterio-venous crossings. Atheromatous plaque formation in the artery at these sites may impinge on the vein lumen, giving a central retinal vein occlusion at the lamina cribrosa or branch vein occlusion at one of the crossings. Thus retinal vein occlusion is most common in patients with a predisposition to the development of atheroma, such as those with hypertension, diabetes mellitus, and lipid disorders. Hyperviscosity, papilloedema, and glaucoma also predispose to retinal vein occlusion, the latter because the increased intraocular pressure favours a decrease in blood-flow, therefore increasing the likelihood of venous occlusion.

A 3.5   (a) Partial lipodystrophy—thin face and normal trunk.

       (b) Mesangiocapillary glomerulonephritis.

Recently a prominent association between partial lipodystrophy and mesangiocapillary glomerulonephritis has been reported. This chronic glomerulonephritis, in which glomerular mesangial cells are increased and capillary walls are irregularly thickened, is associated with a variable reduction in serum C3 complement. This is the result of alternate pathway activation and not of deposition in the glomeruli, as it is unrelated to disease activity and may persist after nephrectomy. The fact that renal transplants can become affected by the disease suggests that a continuing systemic abnormality is responsible for the nephritis. The clinical course is usually progressive and there is no effective treatment.

A 3.6   (a) Diabetic retinopathy.

       (b) (i) Peripheral neuropathy;

           (ii) micro- and macro-angiopathy;

           (iii) nephropathy.

The features of diabetic retinopathy may be classified into two groups:

    (1) background retinopathy with microaneurysms, haemorrhages, exudates, and venous changes,

    (2) proliferative retinopathy with new vessel formation, fibrous proliferation, vitreous haemorrhage, and retinal detachment.

Microaneurysms in the retina occur most frequently in diabetes mellitus but occasionally may be seen in retinal vein closure, Coat's disease, glaucoma, hypertension, pernicious anaemia, and other systemic disease. In diabetes they consist of dilatation on the venous side of the capillary circulation, probably as a result of capillary closure. Exudates may be hard or soft, the latter being the result of capillary closure causing retinal ischaemia.

Haemorrhages in diabetes may be:
(1) small and round, located in the minor muscular layer and thus unable to spread, because the cells are arranged so compactly;

(2) flame-shaped, because they are located in innermost layer of the retina and reflect the nerve fibre distribution;

(3) blot, because the haemorrhage is pre-retinal and held adjacent to the retina by its internal limiting membrane.

Neovascularization indicates a poor prognosis for retinopathy. The new vessels most commonly arise from a retinal vein at the posterior pole or from the surface of the optic disc. They start as delicate lace-like vessels (rete mirabile) which become more fibrous with connective tissue surrounding them. Blood vessels may adhere to the posterior face of the vitreous body. If the vitreous body contracts, vitreous haemorrhages may occur and the retina may be dragged forward causing retinal detachment.

A 3.7   (a) Tuberculous cervical lymphadenitis.

(b) Histology of gland biopsy.

Bovine tuberculosis is usually acquired following the ingestion of unpasteurized milk. The primary lesion may occur in the tonsils and give rise to a glandular component in the cervical lymph glands. The draining regional nodes are termed scrofula. With milk infection the primary lesion may also occur in the intestine, with a glandular component in the mesenteric lymph nodes and sometimes causing secondary abdominal infection. Bovine tuberculosis is unusual since the advent of TB-free herds.

At present tuberculous cervical lymphadenitis is seen most frequently among the Asian immigrant population. In these patients it is almost certainly due to secondary infection rather than a primary complex.Although there is rarely overt evidence of tuberculosis elsewhere, the prolonged course of medical therapy recommended in these patients is based on the principle that the glands form only part of the total problem.

Diagnosis is normally established by gland biopsy. Histological examination of the excised gland is very accurate, culture of either fresh lymph nodes or aspirated pus being considerably less successful. Identification of acid-fast bacilli on a smear preparation of lymph nodes or pus is even less successful.

A 3.8   (a) Posterior communicating artery.

      (b) (i) Subarachnoid haemorrhage;

            (ii) sudden painful third nerve palsy.

Berry aneurysms of the major intracranial arteries arise at sites of congenital defects in the muscular coat. Routine autopsies show an increasing incidence of these lesions with age and also an association with coarctation of the aorta and congenital polycystic disease of the kidney. About 90 per cent involve the circle of Willis, the most common site being at the point of junction of the posterior communicating artery and the internal carotid artery. Spontaneous rupture causes subarachnoid haemorrhage.

    Lateralizing neurological signs may help localize the site of bleeding. Unilateral oculomotor paresis with ptosis, diplopia, and mydriasis suggests that the bleeding source is from the posterior communicating–internal carotid artery junction, which is close to the oculomotor nerve as it passes from the posterior to the middle fossa. Bilateral paresis of the extremities suggests the site of bleeding is near the anterior cerebral anterior communicating artery junction with extension of bleeding into both frontal lobes. Severe hemiparesis and hemianaestheia suggest bleeding from a middle cerebral aneurysm in the sylvian fissure.

A 3.9   (a) Syphilitic aortic aneurysm.

      (b) Paralysis of right recurrent laryngeal nerve.

Syphilitic aortitis gives rise to the three A's, namely, angina pectoris, aortic incompetence, and aneurysm of the aorta. Negative Wasserman's reaction does not exclude syphilitic aortitis–it is positive in no more than 85 per cent of cases. Ascending arch aneurysms are normally asymptomatic, but may produce some pain in the right side of the chest or back, or swelling of the face or arms, or a feeling of engorgement there on stooping. Right recurrent laryngeal nerve involvement at first produces abductor paralysis, and then complete paralysis, giving rise to the 'bovine' cough without any explosive character. Stridor may be present, particularly during sleep. Characteristic signs include unilateral (right-sided) clubbing, lower blood-pressure on the right side, ringing aortic second sound, systolic and early diastolic murmurs, and diminished breath sounds at the apex of the right lung.

A 3.10   (a) Carpopedal spasm.

      (b) Alkalotic tetany due to hysterical hyperventilation.

Carpopedal spasm results in flexion of the metacarpal joints and adduction of the thumbs across the palms and is an important manifestation of tetany. The principal causes of tetany are hypocalcaemia and alkalosis. A reduction in both serum-ionized and protein-bound calcium occurs in vitamin D deficiency states and hypoparathyroidism. Alkalosis, either respiratory or metabolic, increases protein-bound calcium resulting in a reduction of serum concentration of ionized calcium.

A 3.11   (a) Fat atrophy from insulin injections.

(b) Blood sugar.

Fat atrophy in diabetics usually occurs as a result of insulin injections. This problem is less frequent when highly purified insulin is used. As the most suitable sites of injection are areas which are usually covered in public by some form of clothing, such as outer aspects of thighs, buttocks, and lower abdomen then these areas may reveal fat atrophy and suggest a cause of the coma.

A 3.12   (a) Tylosis (the green colour is unusual).

(b) Carcinoma of the oesophagus.

Tylosis is a rare, genetically determined hyperkeratosis of the palms and soles, which is associated with a marked tendency to develop carcinoma of the oesophagus. Other causes of hyperkeratosis of the soles are keratoderma blenorrhagicum, chronic inorganic arsenic poisoning, and vitamin A deficiency. Psoriasiform lesions of secondary syphilis may also occur on the soles and palms.

A 3.13   (a) Hypopituitarism.

(b) (i) Pituitary tumour;

(ii) post-partum pituitary necrosis.

The most common cause of hypopituitarism in adults is pituitary tumour, particularly chromophobe adenoma. Very severe hypopituitarism is most frequently caused by post-partum necrosis of the gland. Granulomatous disease, internal carotid aneurysms, meningitis, basal skull fracture, septic cavernous sinus thrombosis, hypothalamic space occupying lesions are infrequent causes of pituitary insufficiency. Symptoms related to gonadotrophin deficiency are usually the first to appear in hypopituitarism, followed by those related to thyroid and adrenocortical failure. However, there is no set pattern and non-specific symptoms such as anorexia without cachexia, weakness, indifference, and fatigue frequently occur. As one expects, the speed of onset of pituitary insufficiency depends on the nature and size of the underlying lesion.

A 3.14   (a) Angular kyphosis (gibbus).

(b) Pott's disease (tuberculous spondylitis).

The most serious form of bone tuberculosis is Pott's disease because spinal compression may develop. The focus usually originates in the anterior aspect of the vertebral body near an intervertebral disc. As the infection proceeds it may erode the cortex, destroy the intervertebral disc, and affect the adjacent vertebral body. Rarefaction and destruction of adjacent areas of two vertebral bodies, loss of the intervening disc space, and vertebral collapse are typical of Pott's disease (Fig. 3A) but may also be caused by other organisms, especially staphyloccoci, gram-negative enterobacteria, and fungi. The thoracic, thoraco-lumbar, cervical, and lumbosacral areas are involved in order of decreasing frequency.

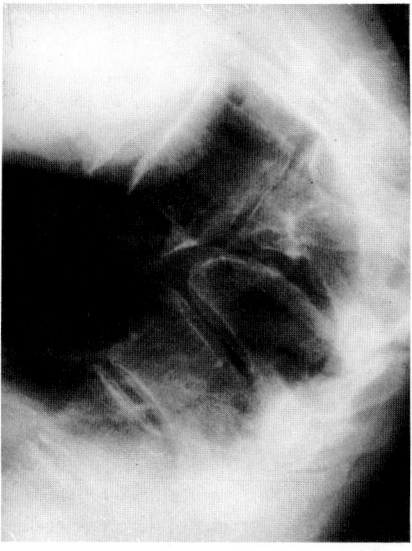

Fig. 3A
Pott's disease with destruction of adjacent areas of two vertebral bodies, loss of intervening disc space, and vertebral collapse.

(i) Infection, particularly streptococcus and tuberculosis;

(ii) drugs, such as sulphonamides and oral contraceptives;

(iii) sarcoidosis;

(iv) chronic inflammatory bowel disease.

Erythema nodosum is probably the result of a hypersensitivity vasculitis usually involving the skin and subcutaneous tissue of the lower leg. The lesions are red, tender, and indurated, gradually becoming darker in colour and finally resembling bruises. This process may resolve in a few days or last several weeks. No cause for erythema nodosum may be found. The pattern of known causes varies geographically, e.g. in Scandinavia tuberculosis or sarcoidosis is the most common underlying disorder, in California it is coccidioidomycosis, and in Massachusetts it is streptococcal pharyngitis.

A 3.16 (a) Pulmonary embolus.

(b) $S_1 Q_3 T_3$ pattern with inversion of T-waves in right ventricular leads; $S_1 T_3$ or T_3 with right ventricular T-wave inversion; $S_1 Q_3 T_3$ with right bundle-branch block.

Pathognomonic electrocardiographic changes probably occur in less than 10 per cent of patients (Fig 3B). They are normally seen with large emboli and the changes are apt to disappear within a few days. Apart from sinus tachycardia, the ECG may remain completely normal. The three patterns mentioned above are the result of acute right ventricular strain. Occasionally only T-wave inversion in the right ventricular chest leads or right bundle branch block is found. Right ventricular hypertrophy is not seen in acute pulmonary embolism. Rhythm changes and P-wave changes are uncommon.

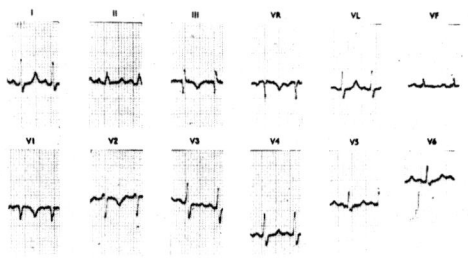

Fig. 3B
$S_1 Q_3 T_3$ with right ventricular T-wave inversion in ECG of patient who developed a large pulmonary embolus.

A 3.17 (a) Iritis.

(b) Sarcoidosis; tuberculosis; ankylosing spondylitis; rheumatoid arthritis; inflammatory bowel disease; toxoplasmosis; syphilis; Behçet's disease.

Dilatation of the ciliary blood vessels in the eye, with blurring and change of colour of the iris characterizes acute iritis. The pupil is always affected, often becoming small and usually irregular in a small part of its margin. There is usually interference with the pupillary reflexes. Chronicity results in a decrease in ciliary injection and the development of adhesions (synechiae) between the iris and lens, or between iris and cornea.

A 3.18   (a) Sclerotic lumbar vertebra with normal IVP.

(b) Paget's disease; osteosclerotic secondary; or reticulosis.

Three types of bone change may be found in Paget's disease:

1. Lytic areas suggesting active disease;

2. New bone growing from the cortex into the medulla and enlarging the bone, giving coarse, irregular trabeculations;

3. Diffuse increase of density with residual bone enlargement, denoting inactivity of the lesion.

The bones most frequently affected are the pelvis, femur, tibia, lower part of the spine, and the skull. The differential diagnosis includes a variety of metastatic tumours (especially prostate) which cause an increase in bone density.

A 3.19   (i)   Trauma;

(ii) hypoalbuminaemia, usually due to cirrhosis of the liver or nephrotic syndrome;

(iii) febrile illness.

Leuconychia is the presence of whiteness of the whole of the nail or of white flecks or bands. The commonest cause of white fleck or bands is minor local injury. White transverse bands initially starting near the lunula, progressing with nail growth towards the free margin, and sometimes associated with shallow transverse ridges or grooves are called Beau's line. They may occur in any febrille illness. In undulant fever, as in brucellosis and lymphomas, successive white bands may be related to periods of fever. In hypoalbuminaemia the whiteness is not in the nail itself but in the nail bed and therefore does not grow with the nail plate.

A 3.20   (a) Vitiligo with hyperpigmentation.

(b) Auto-immune Addison's disease.

In vitiligo, pigment cells present at birth are destroyed. Pigment may be lost from exposed areas, particularly the face and dorsal aspects of the hands, surrounding body orifices, in the axillae and genitalia, at sites of pressure and

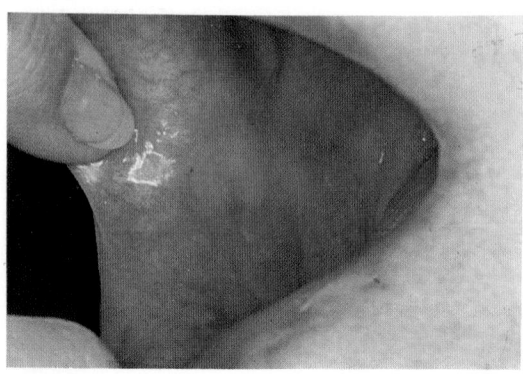

Fig. 3C
Buccal pigmentation
in Addison's disease.

trauma. Vitiligo is transmitted as a dominant trait. Its incidence is increased about tenfold in patients with auto-immune disease and melanomas. In Addison's disease cortisol deficiency results in increased secretion of ACTH and MSH and consequent mucocutaneous accumulation of melanin. The buccal mucosa may have brown, blue, or grey spots (Fig. 3C). As hyper-pigmentation develops, vitiligo tends to occur, with lightening in some areas and darkening in others. This process may also occur in hyperthyroidism.

PAPER 4

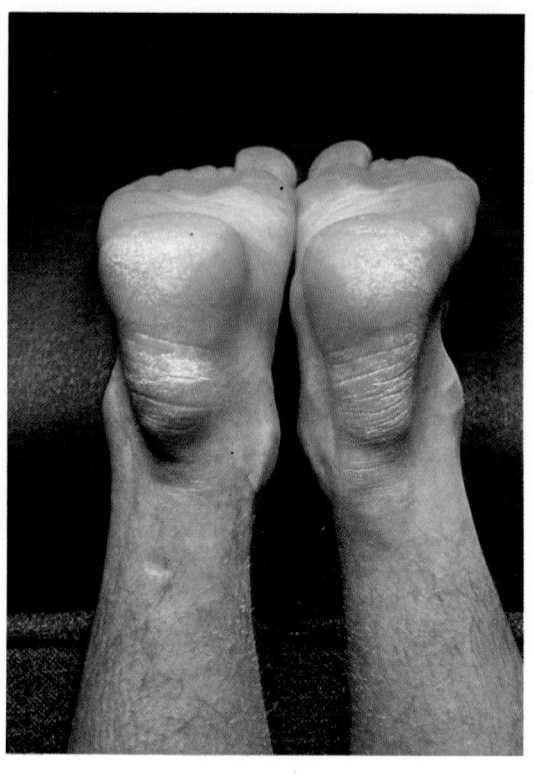

Q 4.1   (a) What is the abnormal physical sign?

(b) What is the most likely cause of this abnormality?

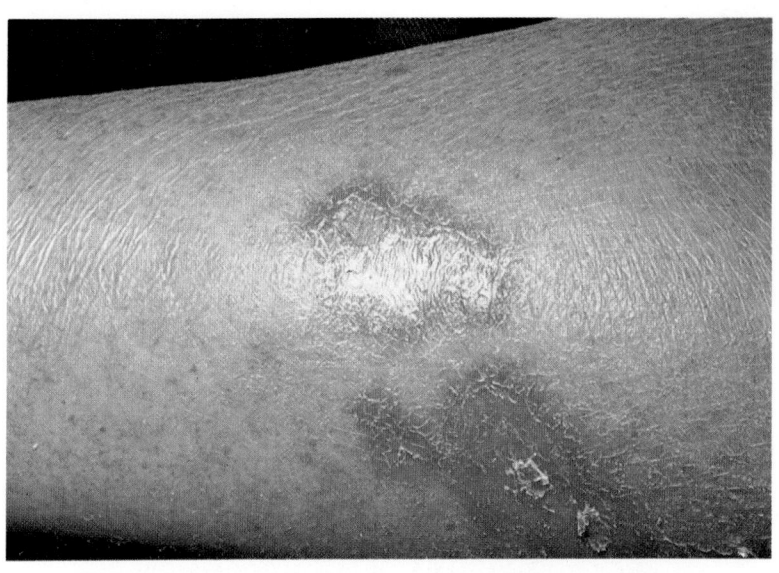

Q 4.2   This lady presented with weight loss and thirst.

    (a) What is the rash?

    (b) What is the most likely cause of the weight loss?

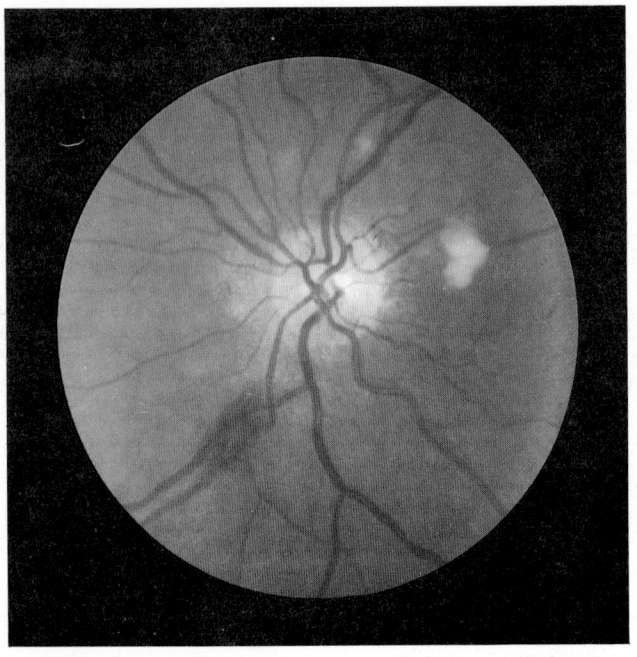

Q 4.3   This patient has had a false-positive Wasserman reaction for three years.

(a) Name the abnormalities in the fundus.

(b) What is the most likely diagnosis?

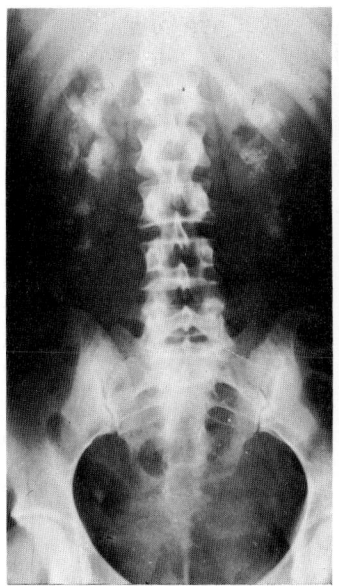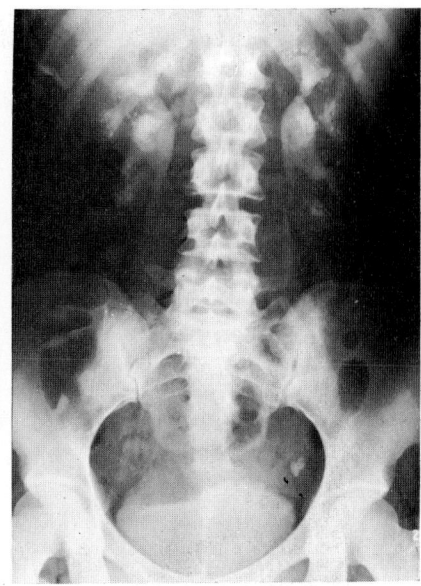

Q 4.4   This patient complained of pain in his feet and inability to get up from the toilet. An IVP was performed, although blood urea was normal. Control film is shown on the left.

(a) What is the abnormality visible on the X-rays?

(b) What is the most likely cause of this patient's foot pain?

(c) How would you treat this patient's foot pain?

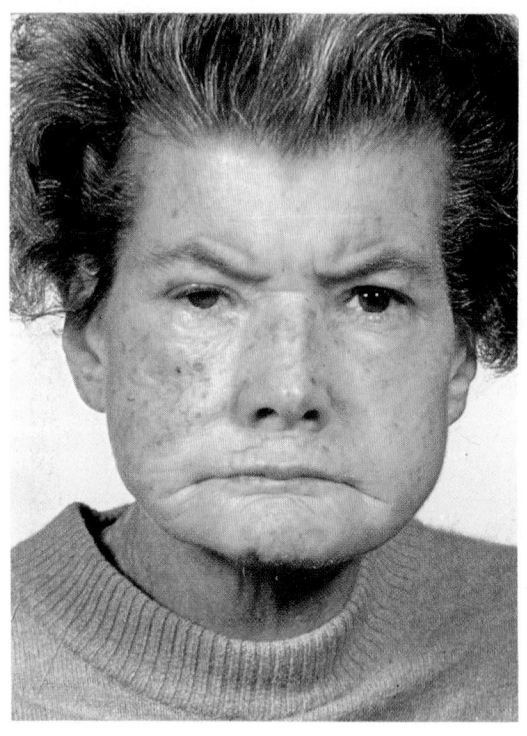

Q 4.5 (a) Name two abnormalities.

(b) Name the two most common, fatal complications of this disorder.

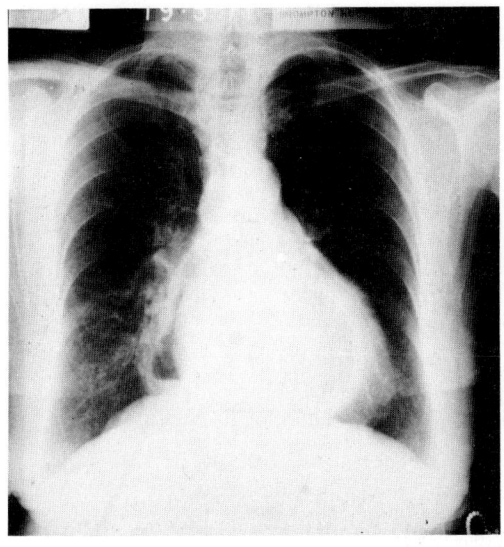

Q 4.6   (a) What is the most likely cause of this X-ray appearance?

          (b) What confirmatory investigation would you always do?

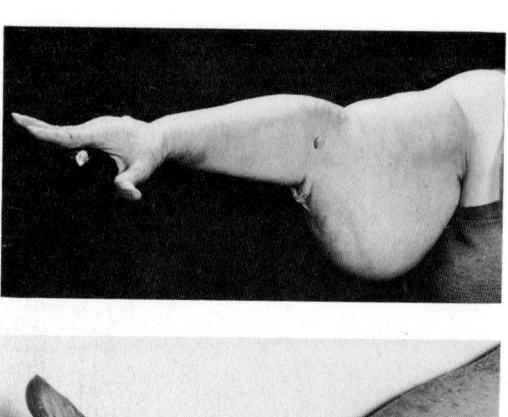
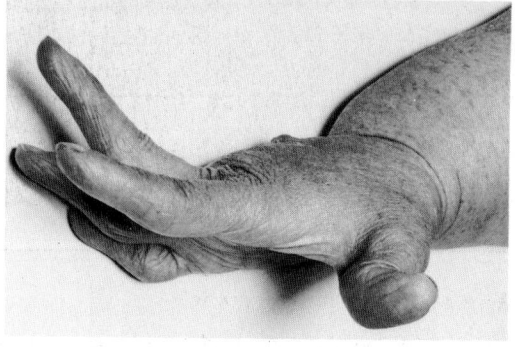

Q 4.7   (a) What is the diagnosis?

   (b) Name four characteristic physical signs of this disorder.

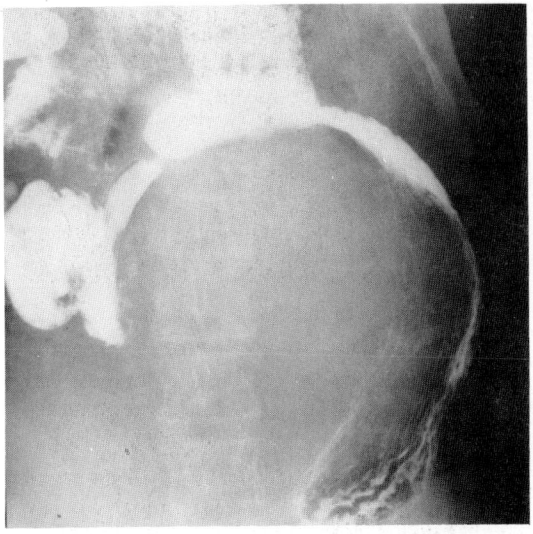

Q 4.8   (a) What is the most likely diagnosis?

(b) What would be the most useful investigation to support the diagnosis?

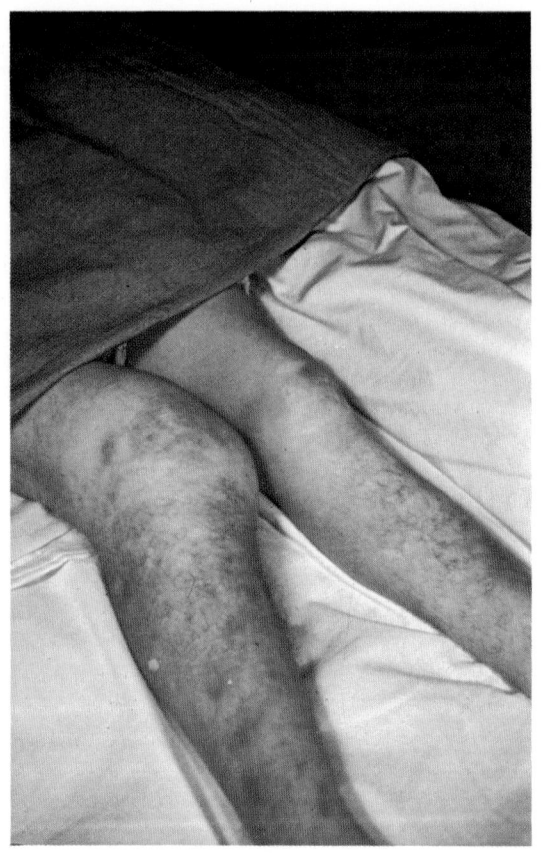

Q 4.9 This patient complained of unsteadiness, but not of pain.

(a) What is the major physical sign?

(b) Name the two most common causes of this abnormality in Britain.

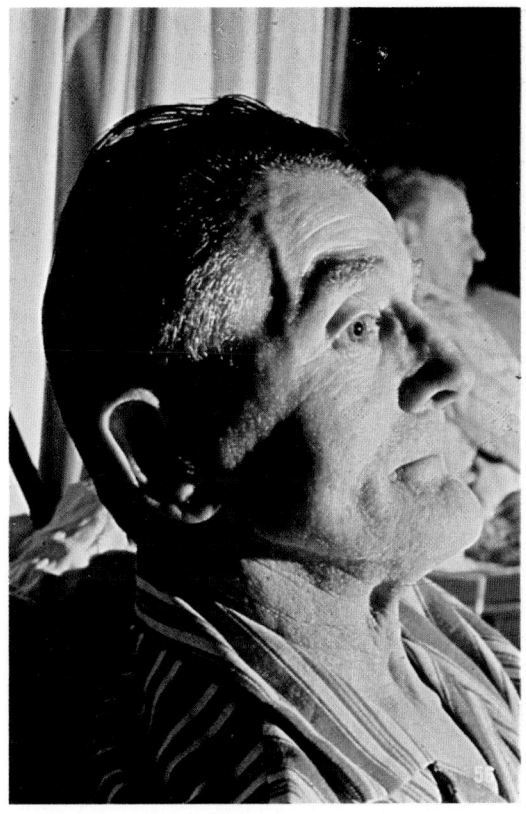

Q 4.10   This patient presented with a severe headache.
          What treatment would you immediately initiate?

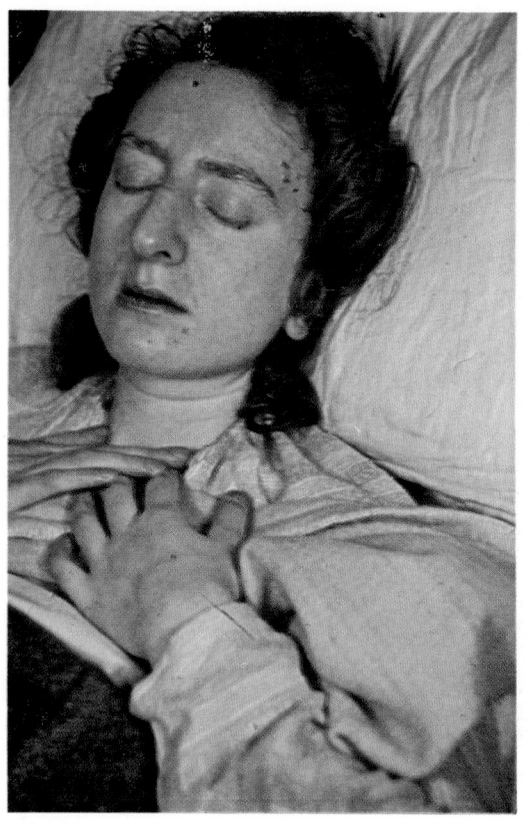

Q 4.11   (a) Name two abnormal physical signs.

(b) What are the two most likely diagnoses?

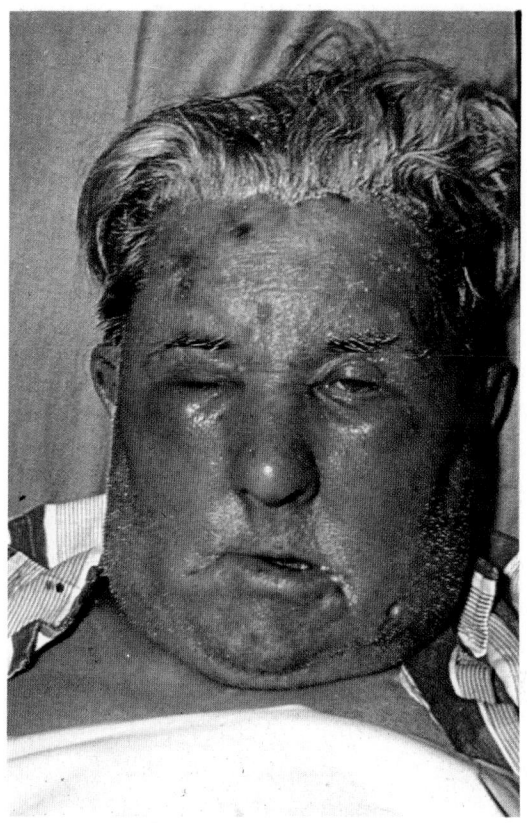

Q 4.12   (a) What is the diagnosis?

(b) What is the cause of this disorder?

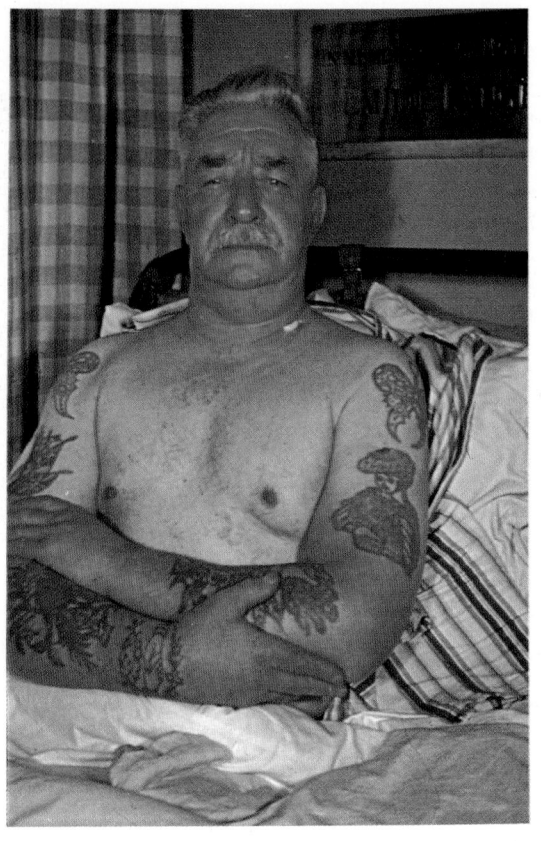

Q 4.13   (a) What is the diagnosis?

(b) What is the most common cause of this problem?

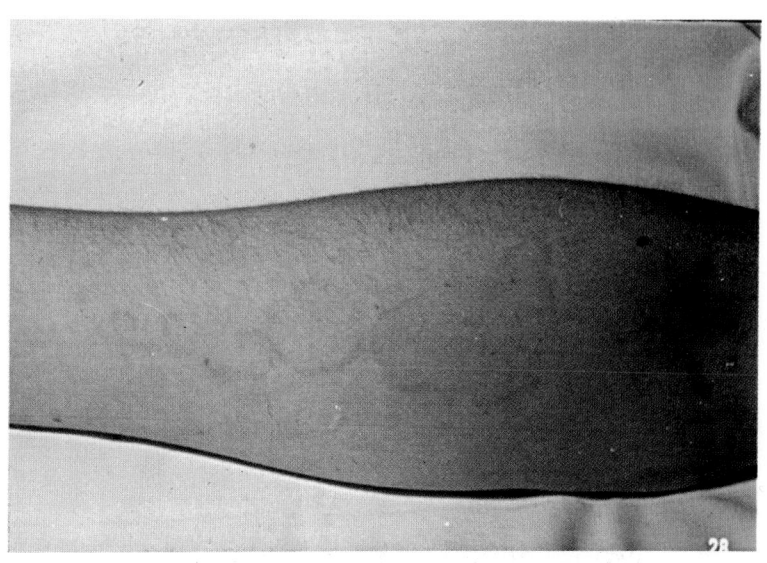

Q 4.14   This patient presented with involuntary movements.

(a) Name the abnormal physical sign.

(b) What two initial investigations would you do to support your diagnosis?

(c) What is the most serious complication of this condition?

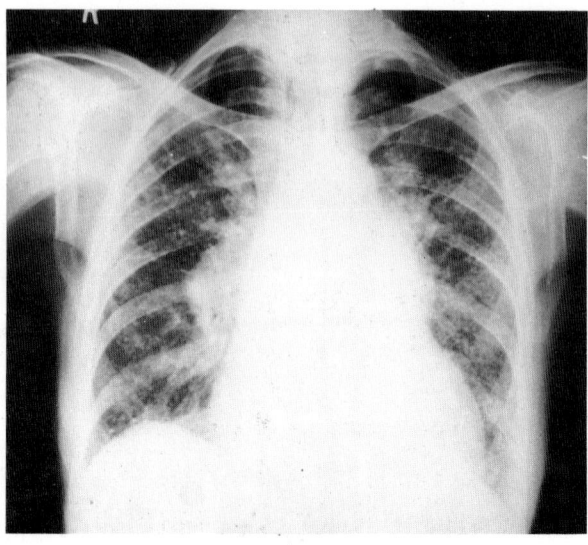

Q 4.15 This patient presented with progressive dyspnoea on exertion over the previous year. Clubbing was present.

(a) Name two abnormalities visible on this chest X-ray.

(b) What is the most likely diagnosis?

(c) How would you confirm your diagnosis?

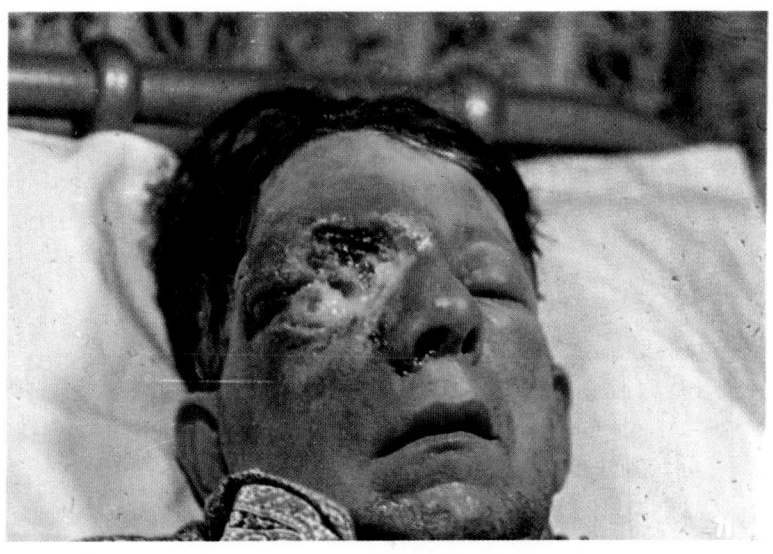

Q 4.16   (a) What is the differential diagnosis?

(b) What single investigation would you like to do?

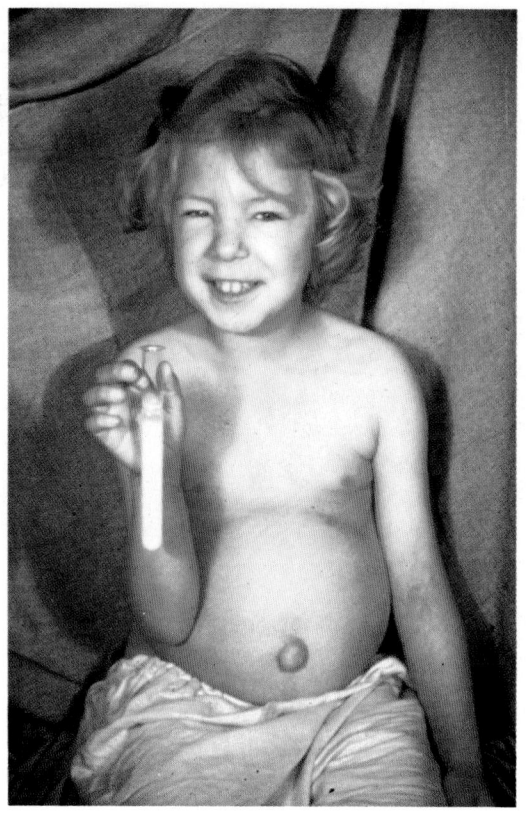

Q 4.17 The patient is holding a test tube of urine to which salicylsulphonic acid has been added.

What is the most likely cause of this disorder in this patient?

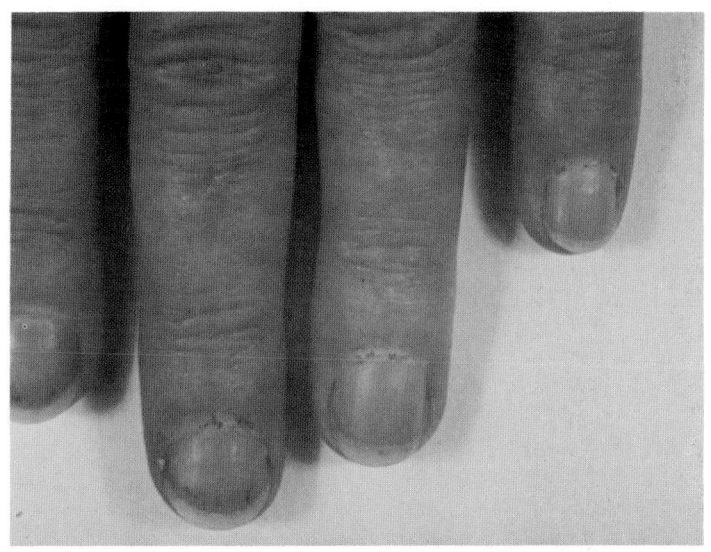

Q 4.18   (a) What are these lesions?

(b) What is the most important initial investigation required to elicit a cause of these lesions?

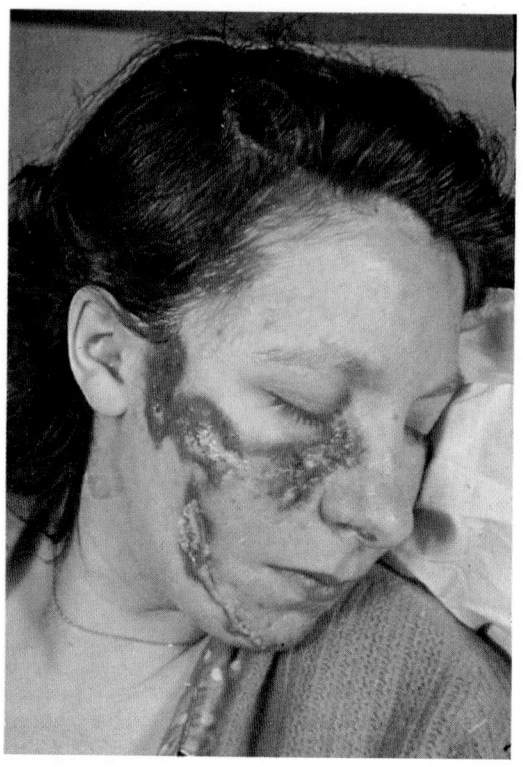

Q 4.19 A 26-year-old woman presented with this lesion, which progressed within one week into a destructive burrowing ulcer.

(a) What is this lesion?

(b) Name two systemic disorders which may be associated with the lesion.

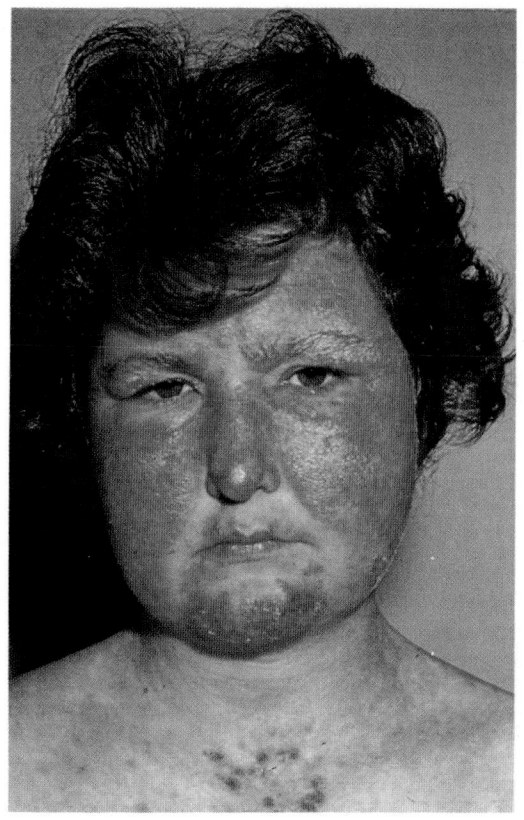

Q 4.20   This patient returned from Spain two weeks previously.

      (a) What is the diagnosis?

      (b) Name three drugs which may induce this rash.

A 4.1   (a) Tendon xanthoma.

(b) Type II hyperlipoproteinaemia.

Tendon xanthomas are found particularly in the Achilles, plantar, patellar, and digital extensor tendons of the hands and are best seen when the tendon is put under tension.

Type II hyperlipoproteinaemia, inherited as a Mendelian dominant trait, is characterized by increased concentration of low-density lipoprotein of normal composition. Tendon xanthomas usually do not appear until after puberty, but when present are suggestive of this disorder. Xanthelesma and corneal arcus may also appear but are less clearly associated with lipid disorders.

A 4.2   (a) Necrobiosis lipoidica.

(b) Diabetes mellitus.

Necrobiosis lipoidica is a rare disorder consisting of persistent atrophic plaques, usually on the lower extremities. The lesions begin as darkish red, scaly plaques which are often flat but sometimes have an elevated border. As they gradually enlarge the epidermis and dermis become atrophic and a depressed centre with a yellow cast may develop. The lesions are multiple but not symmetrical. They are seen most frequently on the anterior aspect of the legs but sometimes occur on the forearms and abdomen. Thirty-five per cent of patients with necrobiosis have diabetes mellitus and about a half of non-diabetic patients with the disorder are either pre-diabetic or have relatives with diabetes.

A 4.3   (a) Cotton-wool spot with haemorrhage.

(b) Systemic lupus erythematosus (SLE).

The most common ocular sign in SLE is the cotton-wool spot (containing cytoid bodies) in the superficial layer of the retina. Its presence usually indicates active disease and it disappears during remission. Other retinal changes of SLE include secondary optic atrophy, superficial and deep haemorrhages, and arterial and venous occlusions.

Any febrile disease or immunization is a potential cause of false-positive serological tests for syphilis. False-positive tests of long duration suggest auto-immune disease or dysproteinaemia.

A 4.4   (a) Nephrocalcinosis.

(b) Osteomalacia as a result of renal tubular acidosis.

(c) Correction of the acidosis with alkali.

Renal tubal acidosis may induce renal stones and/or nephrocalcinosis. The hyperchloraemic acidosis is associated with hypercalciuria and a negative calcium balance, which is relatively resistant to vitamin D, but which may respond to treatment with alkali. If severe, the myopathy of osteomalacia may never resolve fully, even when treatment has healed the bones.

A 4.5   (a) (i) Telangiectasiae;

(ii) constriction of skin around mouth.

(b) (i) Renal failure;

(ii) pulmonary fibrosis.

In scleroderma the skin of the face becomes smooth and waxy. Telangiectasiae, with increased or decreased pigmentation, may be seen. The skin around the mouth constricts, restricting lip movement and adequate dental hygiene. The CRST syndrome (calcinosis, Raynaud's phenomenon, sclerodactyly, and telangiectasiae) and the Thibierge–Weissenbach syndrome (diffuse subcutaneous calcification with acrosclerosis) are variants of the cutaneous expression of scleroderma.

Patients with scleroderma have a 50–70 per cent five-year survival. Some patients, particularly those with pulmonary, cardiac, and renal involvement, may progress rapidly to early death. Renal failure is the cause of death in 20–40 per cent of patients. It is rare for patients who suddenly develop malignant hypertension and uraemia to survive longer than four months without renal replacement therapy.

A 4.6   (a) Hiatus hernia with pericardiac shadows and fluid levels.

(b) Lateral chest X-ray.

An opacity, containing a fluid level near the mediastinum suggests a hiatus hernia. However, a similar appearance may result from an intra-pulmonary abscess or gas in the pericardium. The lateral radiograph (Fig. 4A) will illustrate clearly the retrocardiac opacity with a prominent fluid level.

A 4.7   (a) Ehlers–Danlos syndrome.

(b) Cutaneous hyperelasticity; hyperextensibility of joints; easy bruising; atrophic scars and pseudotumours; calcified sub-cutaneous cysts.

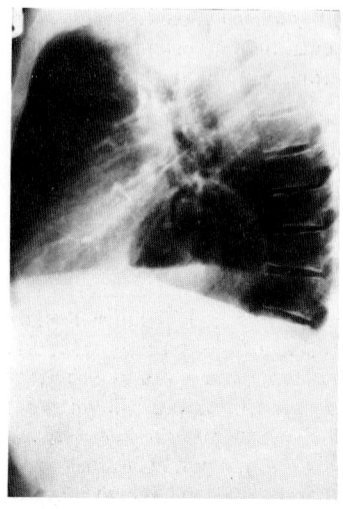

Fig. 4A
Lateral chest X-ray showing a hiatus hernia.

The clinical features of Ehlers–Danlos syndrome are variable because several genetic and incomplete types exist. However the patient is likely to be small, short, and poorly developed. The soft velvety skin is hyperelastic and abnormally fragile. With age this elasticity may be lost and the skin of localized areas, especially about the elbows may hang in loose folds, resembling cutis laxa.

Hyperextensibility of the joints is striking, leading to arthritis and dislocation. Many musculoskeletal abnormalities have been described, as have some internal manifestations, such as aneurysms (aortic and intracranial), spontaneous rupture of the lung, fragility of the bowel, and bleeding tendencies.

A 4.8   (a) Pancreatic cyst.

          (b) Ultrasound.

Swellings in the retroperitoneal space will displace portions of the upper or lower intestinal tract according to its position. A pancreatic cyst will produce displacement of stomach and duodenum without signs of invasion. However, differentiation from other retroperitoneal swellings, including right-sided renal tumours, may be difficult.

Pseudocysts usually lie in the lesser sac and follow pancreatitis (acute or chronic) and trauma. A collection of fluid poorly localized by acutely inflamed tissue may complicate acute pancreatitis. This pseudocyst is quite unlike the well-encapsulated and well-defined retention cyst, which is commonly seen with chronic relapsing pancreatitis and results from intrapancreatic obstruction. Pseudocysts, complicating acute pancreatitis, often heal spontaneously, whereas in chronic pancreatitis they persist indefinitely. The development of a pseudocyst may be confirmed simply and safely by ultrasound.

A 4.9   (a) Charcot joint (with knee swelling and deformity).

(b) (i) Diabetes;

(ii) late syphilis.

At present, diabetes is the most common cause of Charcot joints in Britain. They also occur in other neurological disorders, such as syringomyelia and late syphilis. With the latter disorder, the Charcot joint develops as a result of destruction of sensory neurons in tabes dorsalis. It often appears in burnt-out cases with normal blood and spinal serology. The Charcot joint, which swells painlessly with trauma, is usually confined to a single weight-bearing joint, but in syringomyelia may occur in the upper limbs. The joint becomes hyper-mobile and loses its contour. Gradually the joint surface disintegrates and gross deformity results (Fig. 4B).

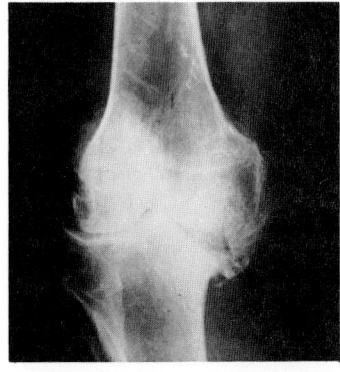

Fig. 4B
Charcot joint with gross degenerative disease and deformity.

A 4.10   High doses of corticosteroids.

Temporal arteritis most often affects the branches of the external carotid artery. When the temporal artery is affected it may be tender, thickened, and nodular and is usually pulseless. The most feared complication of cranial arteritis is acute blindness, which may be permanent. This results from ophthalmic or ciliary artery involvement and can be prevented by immediate therapy with steroids. This treatment should not be delayed while awaiting a temporal artery biopsy which will still be diagnostic shortly after the initiation of therapy.

A 4.11   (a) (i) Central cyanosis;

(ii) clubbing.

(b) (i) Congenital heart disease;

(ii) anoxic cor pulmonale.

When central cyanosis is severe and chronic, polycythaemia and digital clubbing may accompany it. Right to left intracardiac shunts (such as Fallot's tetralogy and Eisenmerger complex) and chronic lung disease with intrapulmonary shunting are the commonest causes of chronic cyanosis. The rate of development and degree of clubbing are extremely variable.

A 4.12   (a) Erysipelas.

(b) Group A streptococci.

Erysipelas usually presents with the sudden onset of fever and a shaking chill. It frequently involves the face and head but may involve any part of the body. The lesion usually spreads from a central focus, the advancing edge of the lesion being sharply defined and the skin red, hot, and glistening. Oedema is prominent, especially when the eyelids are involved, and tends to be limited by bony prominences.

A 4.13   (a) Superior vena caval obstruction with oedematous face and upper limbs, with engorgement of the veins on the chest and neck.

(b) Bronchogenic carcinoma.

Superior vena caval obstruction is usually produced by metastases in mediastinal nodes from bronchogenic carcinoma. The physical signs produced include suffusion and brawny oedema involving the face, neck, and upper limbs, engorged jugular veins without venous pulsation, and dilated veins on chest and upper abdomen, with flow of blood towards the umbilicus. Oesophageal and tracheal constriction may also occur and lead to dysphagia and stridor respectively.

A 4.14   (a) Erythema marginatum.

(b) (i) Throat swab culture;

(ii) antistreptolysin O titre;

(c) Carditis.

Erythema marginatum is a major criterion for the diagnosis of rheumatic fever and occurs in about 5 per cent of patients with this disorder. It almost always coexists with arthritis, chorea, or carditis. The rash consists of pale pink, irregular, serpiginous lines which may become crescentic or circular. It tends to clear from the centre and may leave a brownish area. It occurs on the limbs and trunk, nearly always avoiding the face. The rash is usually transient, occasionally recurring, and rarely chronic.

The important investigations should seek evidence for streptococcal infection, rheumatic fever, disease activity, and carditis. The former may be supported by a high-antistreptolysin O titre or culture of beta-haemolytic streptococci from the throat. ASOT in the region of 200 Todd units suggests a recent haemolytic streptococcal infection but is not proof of rheumatism. Furthermore, a fifth of patients with rheumatic fever may fail to show a rise in ASOT above 200. The e.s.r. is usually very high in active rheumatic fever. Occasionally it may be normal through the entire illness, especially if heart failure develops or in uncomplicated chorea.

The diagnosis of acute carditis may be difficult, especially as prolongation of P–R interval on ECG cannot be regarded as definitive evidence. The diagnosis depends on the recognition of four events which may occur alone or in various combinations: abnormal murmurs, pericardial rub, cardiac enlargement, and congestive cardiac failure.

A 4.15   (a) (i) Diffuse pulmonary shadowing;

(ii) enlarged heart and pulmonary arteries.

(b) Fibrosing alveolitis with pulmonary hypertension.

(c) Lung biopsy.

Diffuse shadowing on the chest X-ray, without evidence of left ventricular failure, may suggest fibrosing alveolitis or some other cause of pulmonary fibrosis.

Fibrosing alveolitis may have an acute or chronic onset. An acute form (Hamman–Rich disease) may lead to death within weeks or months, while the more common chronic type runs a variable course, usually leading to death from respiratory failure, pneumonia, or cor pulmonale. Lung biopsy may confirm the diagnosis and also indicate the likelihood of a favourable response to treatment with steroids.

Diffuse reticular or reticulonodular shadowing is the most common radiological abnormality found in fibrosing alveolitis. Progression may lead to coarsening of the linear shadows and the development of 'honeycombing', together with proximal pulmonary arterial enlargement and cardiomegaly, indicative of pulmonary hypertension.

A 4.16 (a) Lethal midline granuloma/Wegener's granulomatosis.

(b) Biopsy of involved structure.

Lethal midline granuloma is probably a clinical entity with several causes, including syphilis, yaws, leprosy, mucormycosis, carcinoma of nose or paransal sinuses, and lymphomas. Its differentiation from Wegener's granuloma is controversial. In the latter condition granulomas affect blood vessels and cause subsequent necrosis of tissue. Symptoms of nasal discharge and discharge may be present for months prior to development of redness. Then necrosis and progressive loss of facial tissue develops. Diagnosis depends on biopsy of the involved tissue but a cause may not be found until late in the disease or at autopsy.

A 4.17 Nephrotic syndrome due to minimal change glomerulonephritis.

Ninety-five per cent of children under the age of five presenting with nephrotic syndrome have minimal change glomerulonephritis. The proteinuria is highly selective and the urine is free of red cells. Biopsy is rarely necessary and the nephrosis usually responds to steroids, although many may relapse. The aetiology is unknown.

A 4.18 (a) Splinter haemorrhages.

(b) Blood cultures.

The commonest cause of nail haemorrhage is trauma. Splinter haemorrhages are linear, usually longitudinal, and progress towards the free margin with nail growth. They may occur in crops and suggest infective endocarditis but also occur in septicaemias, connective tissue disease, severe anaemia, and any condition with a liability to bleed. Occasionally cervical rib may induce splinters in the ipsilateral hand. Trichiniasis induces transverse linear haemorrhages which do not occur in crops.

The most important investigation is blood culture but microscopy of freshly spun urine may aid diagnosis of infective endocarditis.

A 4.19 (a) Pyoderma gangrenosum.

(b) Ulcerative colitis; polyarthritis (usually seronegative but sometimes seropositive); paraproteinaemia (usually IgA).

Pyoderma gangrenosum begins as a fluctuant pustule or nodule which rapidly ulcerates. The ulcer is destructive and burrowing with an irregular margin and ragged, purple–red, overhanging edge. Lesions may be single or multiple. The course of these lesions is variable but they frequently heal with a cribriform scar.

The aetiology of pyoderma gangrenosum is unknown. In all the diseases associated with it there are disturbed immunological mechanisms and the lesion responds to steroids and other immunosuppressants, suggesting that circulating immune complexes may play an important role.

A 4.20   (a) Systemic lupus erythematosus (SLE) (treated with steroids).

          (b) Hydrallazine, phenylbutazone, diphenylhydantoin, procaineamide, anti-infective agents such as griseoflavin, isoniazid, streptomycin, penicillin, and sulphonamides.

Most patients with idiopathic SLE are women between 10 and 40 years of age. Skin lesions are the first signs in only one-fifth of patients, but are present at some time in more than four-fifths. The lesions centre around the facial and upper chest areas. They are similar to the discoid variety of lupus in some patients but are transient, erythematous, and non-specific in most. The 'butterfly' rash of the nose and malar area presents itself in at least half of those with SLE, although often only for a short time. A history of worsening by sun exposure occurs in one-third or more of cases. Patients with drug-induced disease show slightly different serological abnormalities and are unlikely to develop the two most serious complications, i.e. nephritis and cerebral vasculitis.

PAPER 5

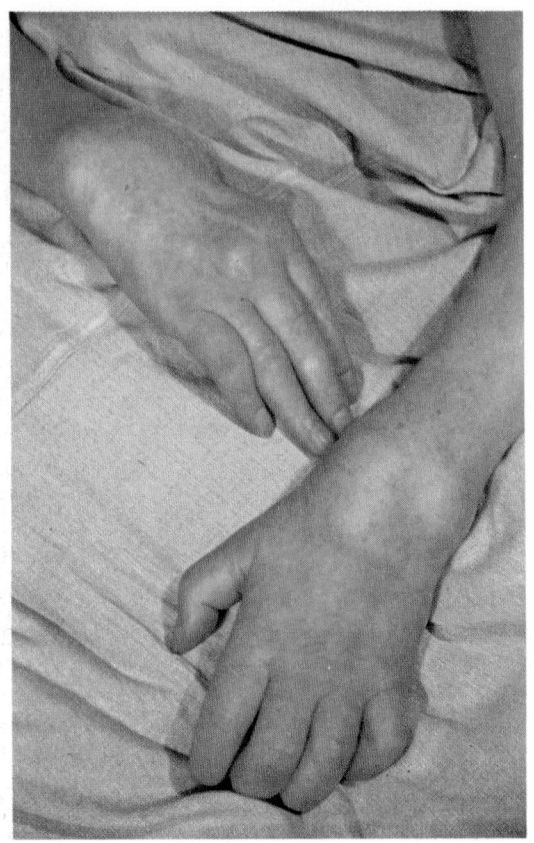

Q 5.1   This patient's hands are painless.

(a) Name two abnormalities visible on this slide.

(b) What is the diagnosis?

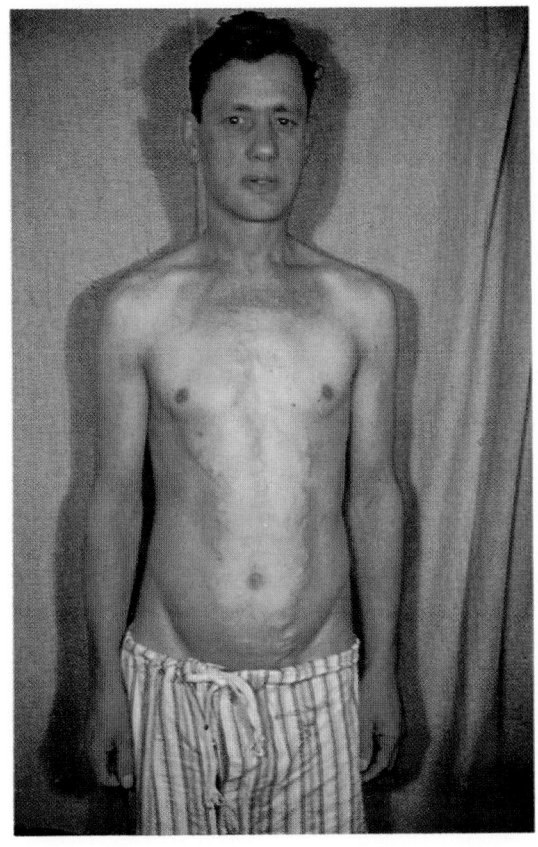

Q 5.2   (a) What physical sign would you elicit on observing this patient?

(b) What is the most likely diagnosis?

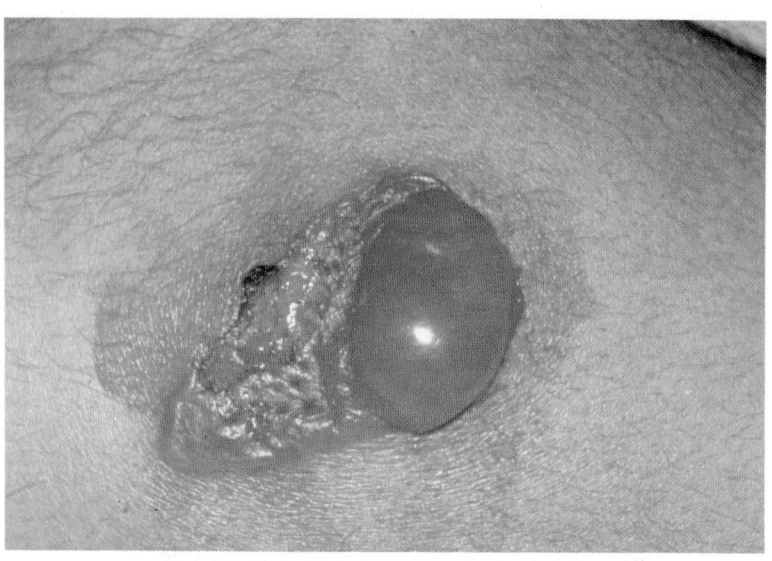

Q 5.3 This 24-year-old patient was admitted, comatose, to the Casualty Department. This physical sign was present on his buttocks.

What is the most likely reason for coma?

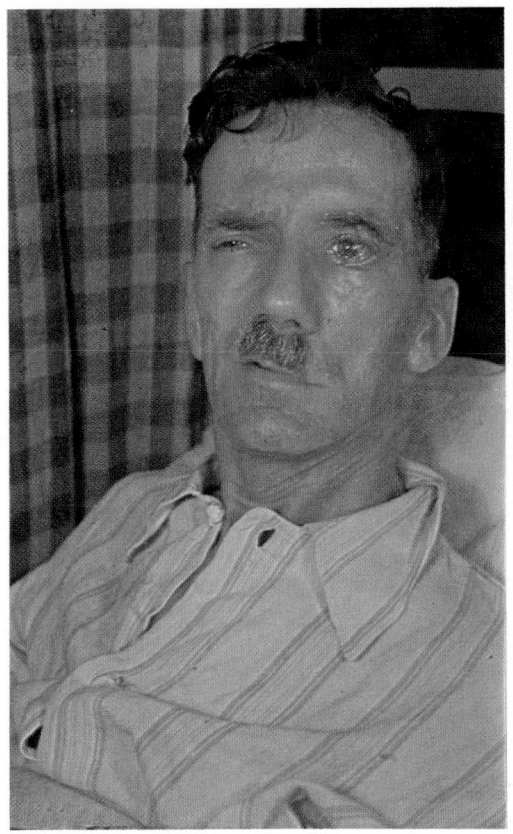

Q 5.4   This patient has right upper limb weakness.

      (a)   Where is the lesion in this patient?

      (b)   What abnormality of the eye (not shown in the slide) should be present in this patient?

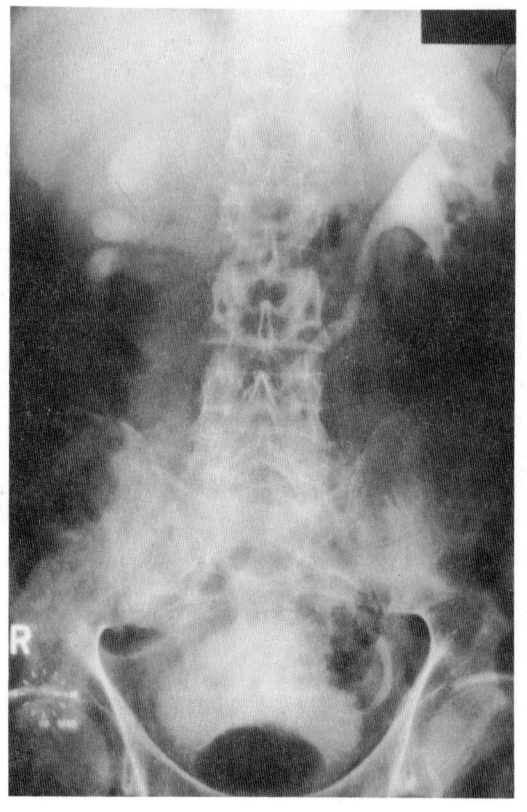

Q 5.5 This patient complained of backache and swelling of his ankles. He had a history of headaches since childhood. An IVP was performed because the patient had renal impairment.

(a) What is the most likely diagnosis?

(b) What drug may have caused this appearance?

(c) How would you treat this patient?

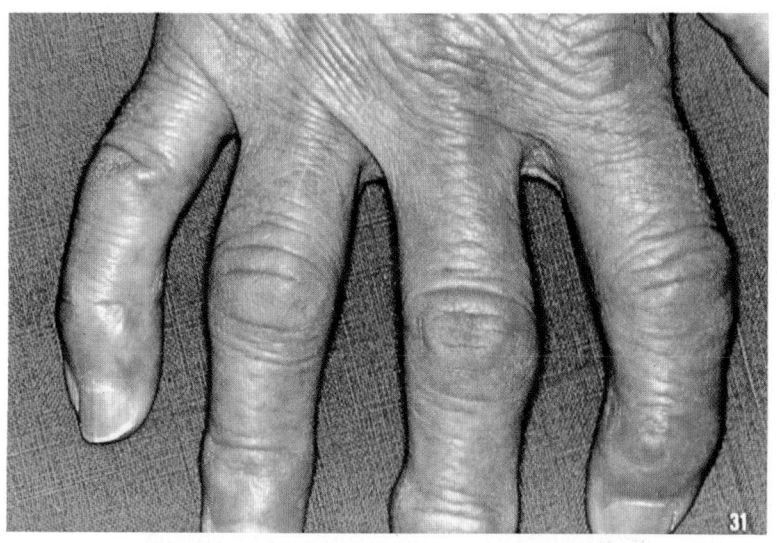

Q 5.6   This patient complained of pain in his knees.

(a) Name two abnormal physical signs.

(b) Which sex is most often affected by these deformities?

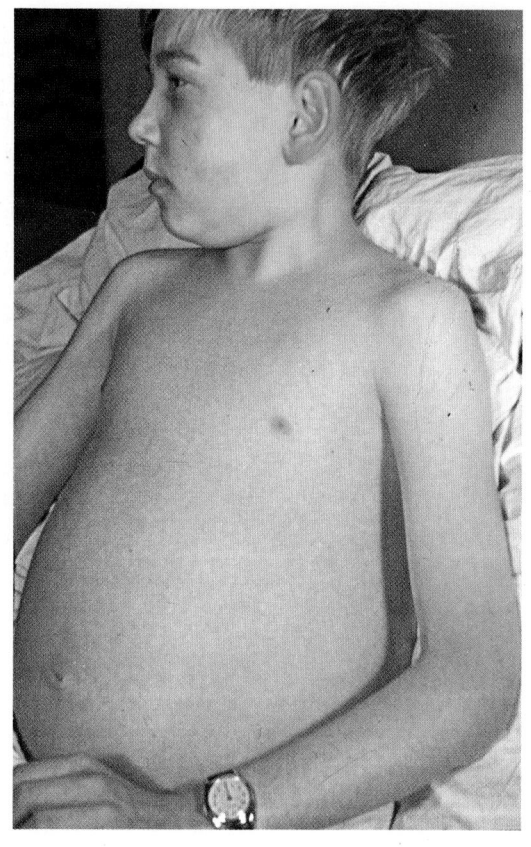

Q 5.7 This patient was able to lie flat without shortness of breath.

What is the most likely diagnosis?

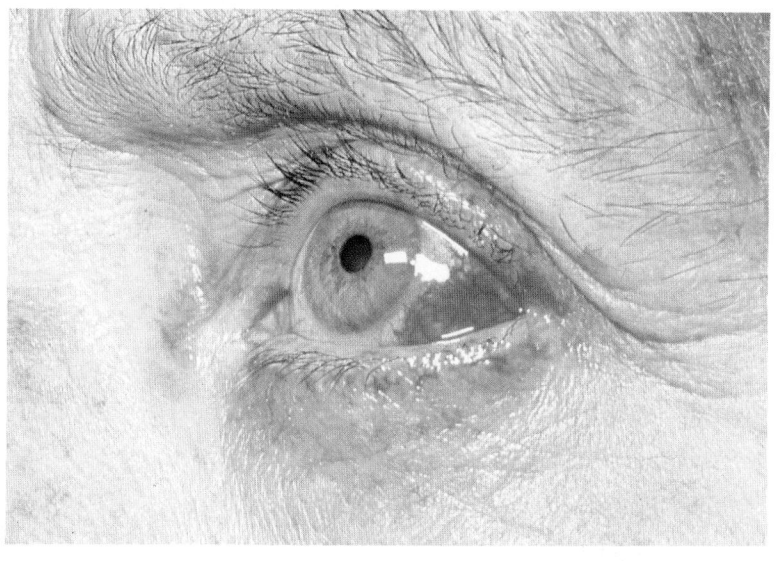

Q 5.8   (a) Name the abnormal physical sign.

(b) What is the most likely cause of this sign?

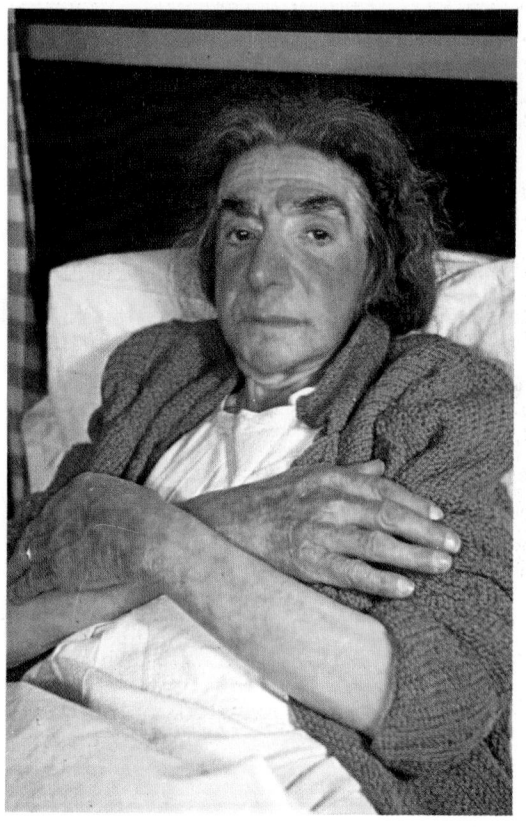

Q 5.9   This alcoholic complained of weakness, irritability, and diarrhoea.

(a) What replacement therapy would you commence to treat the rash?

(b) Name three of the best food sources of this substance.

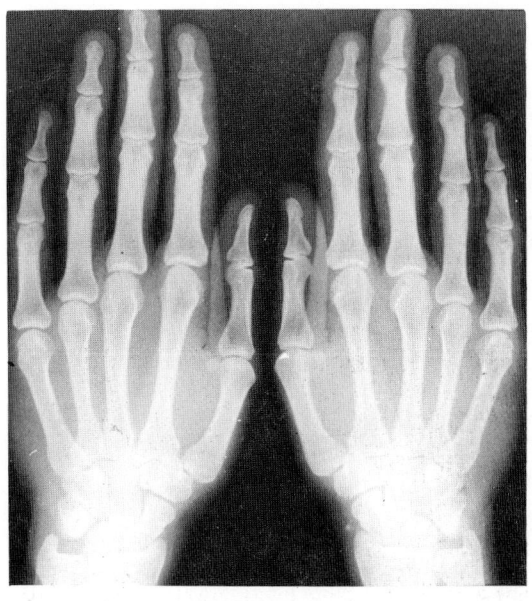

Q 5.10   (a) Name the abnormality visible on this X-ray.

(b) What are the two most likely causes of this picture?

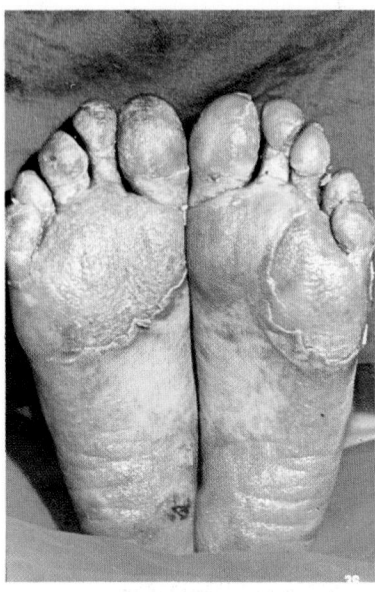 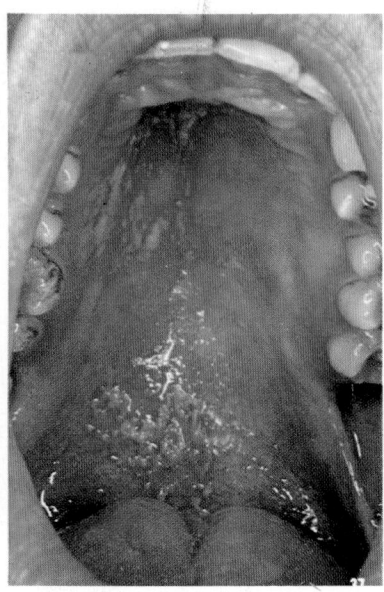

Q 5.11 These two slides are of the same patient.

(a) Name the abnormal physical sign on each slide.

(b) Name four other important manifestations of this disease.

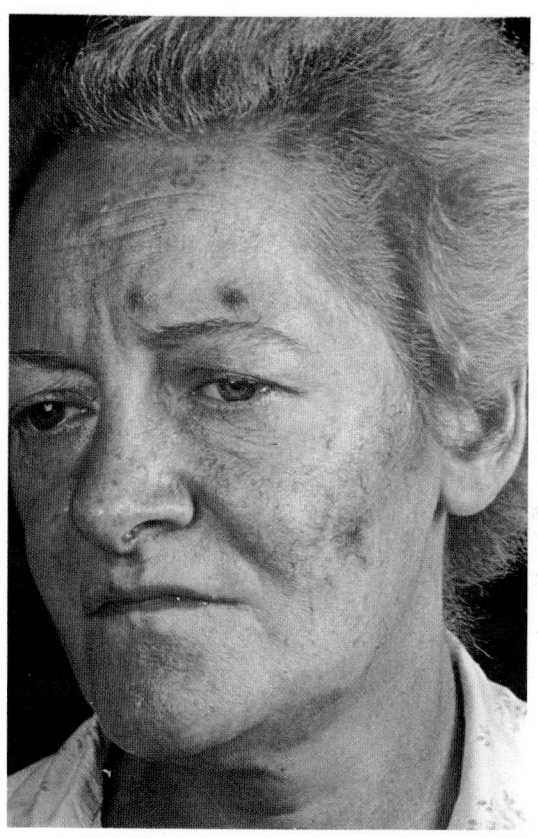

Q 5.12   (a) What are these lesions?

(b) Name four causes of these lesions.

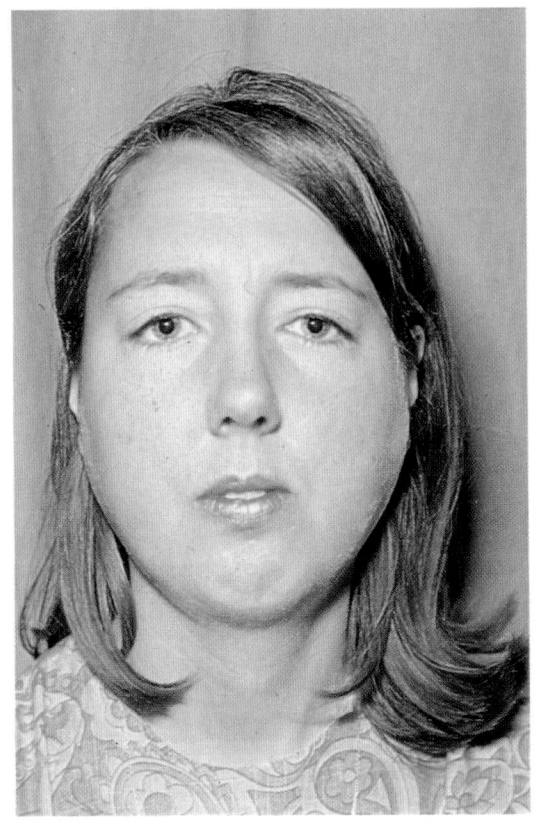

Q 5.13 This sign has been present for two months and been associated with fever.

(a) Name the abnormal physical sign.

(b) What are the three most likely causes of this patient's illness?

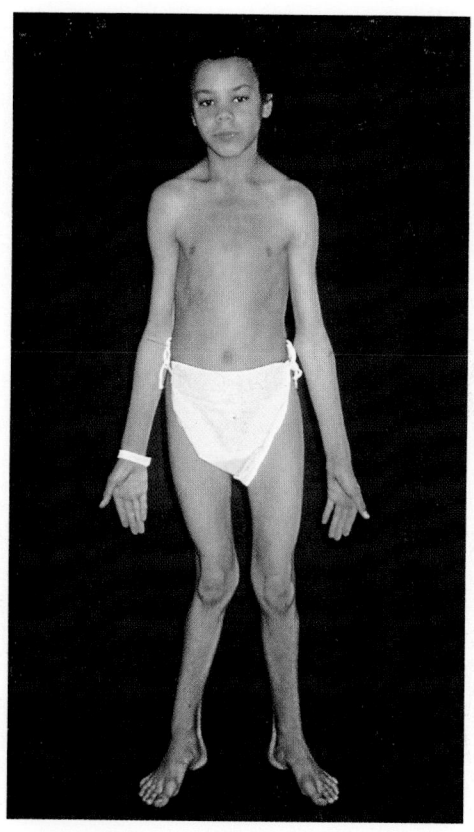

Q 5.14   (a) What is the diagnosis?

(b) Name the three most likely causes of this condition.

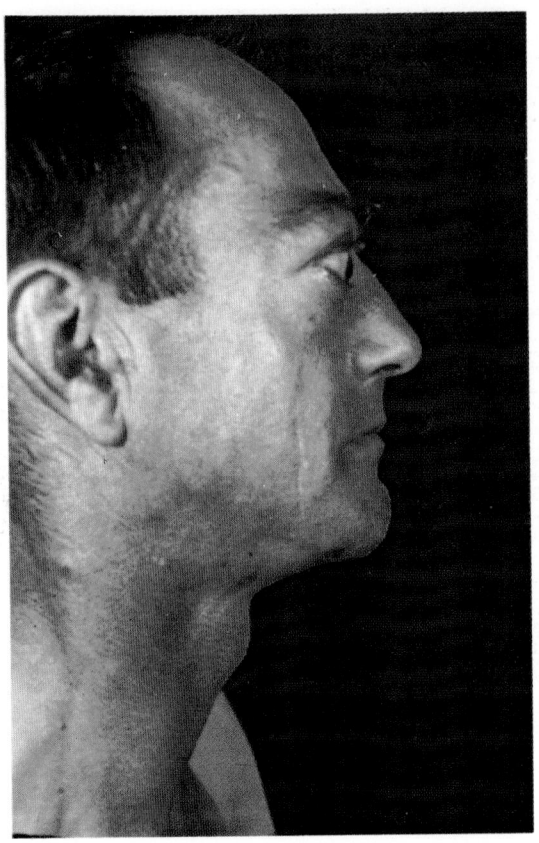

Q 5.15 (a) What is the abnormal physical sign?

(b) What is the most likely cause of this sign?

(c) If this sign were unilateral name two further disorders which should be considered in the differential diagnosis.

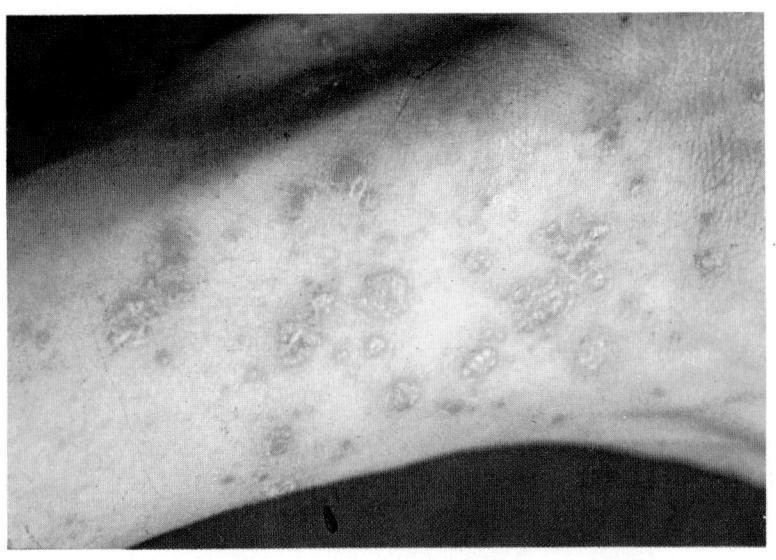

Q 5.16 (a) What is the diagnosis?

(b) What is the average duration of this rash?

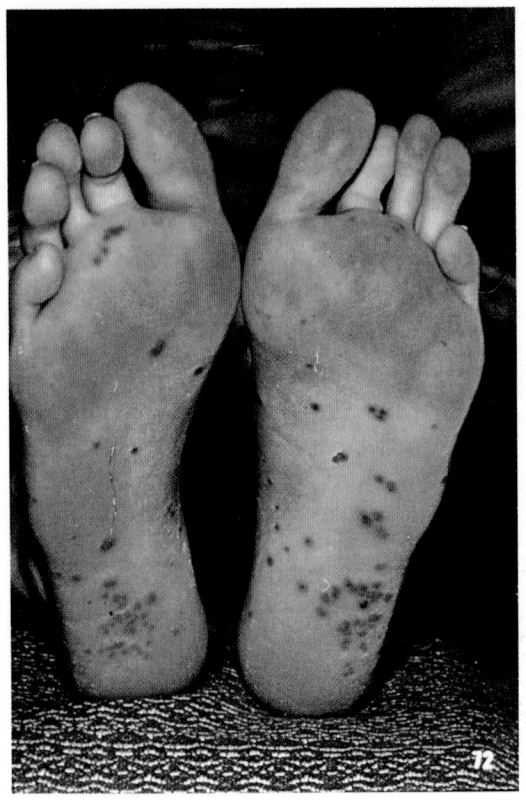

Q 5.17 This thirty-year-old man had intermittent attacks of sweating and palpitations for the previous six months. Then he developed pain in the lower limbs. All serological tests were normal.

(a) Name two abnormal physical signs.

(b) Name two ways in which the kidney may be involved in this disorder.

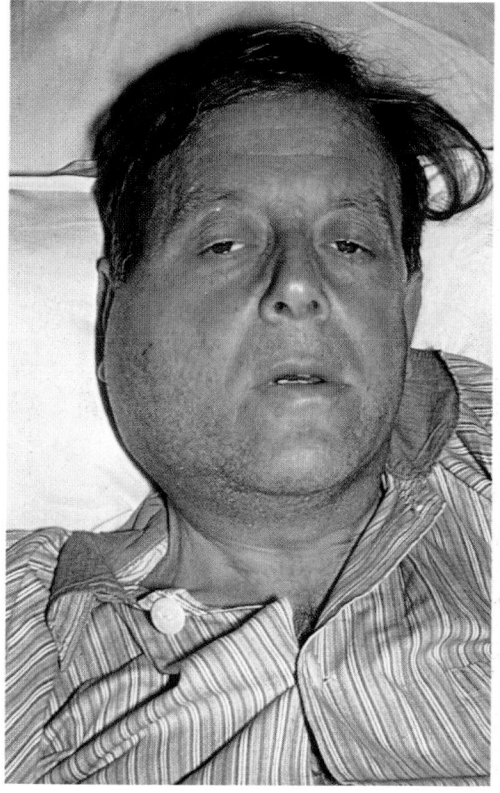

Q 5.18 This patient with renal failure was admitted semi-comatose due to a metabolic acidosis.

(a) What is the abnormal physical sign?

(b) What is the most likely cause of this physical sign?

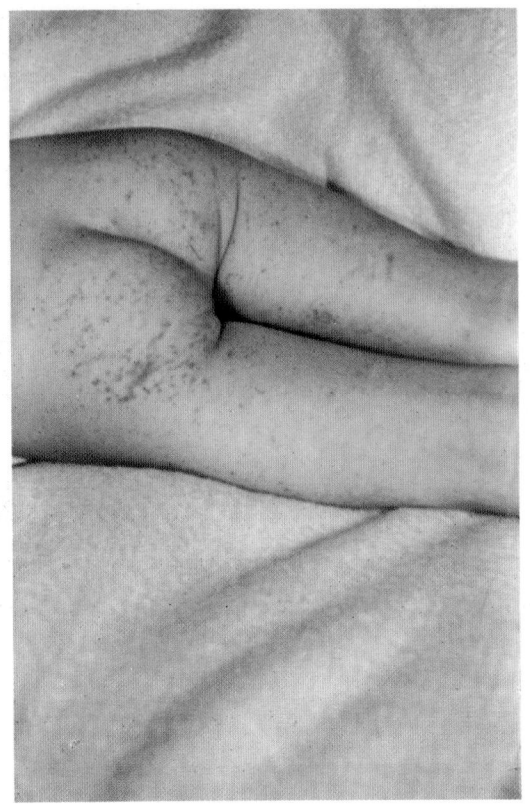

Q 5.19   This 15-year-old patient has proteinuria.

(a) What is the physical sign?

(b) What is the most likely diagnosis?

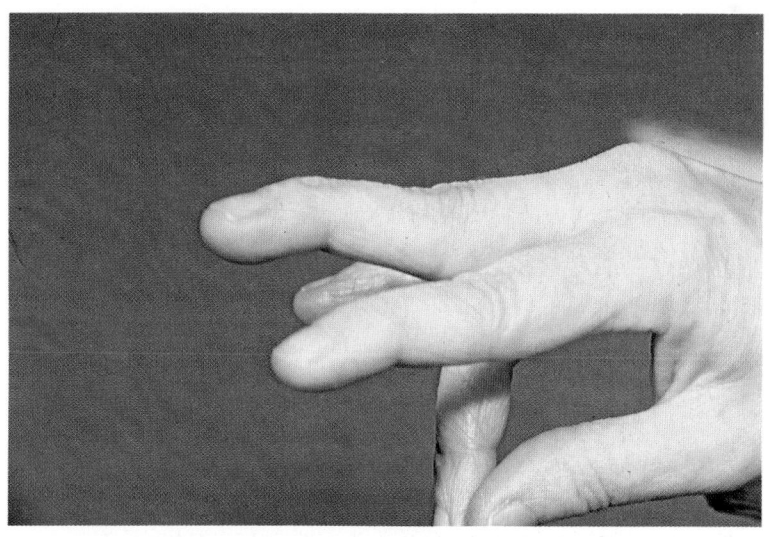

Q 5.20   This psychiatric patient had been treated with drugs for about one
year. He then complained that he was unable to write.

   (a) What is the abnormal physical sign?

   (b) What is the most likely reason for this patient's inability to
write?

A 5.1   (a) (i) Bilateral claw hand;

(ii) Charcot joints of wrists and hands.

(b) Syringomyelia.

Upper limb Charcot arthropathy should always suggest syringomyelia. The diagnosis of syringomyelia is based on (a) segmental sensory loss in the upper limbs affecting pain and temperature sense but sparing touch, (b) amyotrophy, and (c) thoracic scoliosis. The sensory loss results in painless ulcers, injuries (particularly giving Charcot joints), and burns. The most common cause of a bilateral claw hand is syringomyelia due to destruction of the anterior horn cells, but rarer causes are peripheral neuritis and peroneal muscular atrophy.

A 5.2   (a) The direction of blood-flow in the veins.

(b) Inferior vena caval obstruction.

Large veins on the abdominal wall suggest venous obstruction. Venous blood-flow below the umbilicus is normally downwards into the saphenous vein and above the umbilicus is upwards into the thoracic wall veins. In inferior vena caval obstruction the enlarged collateral veins are usually over the lower abdomen and the blood flows upwards, whereas in superior vena caval obstruction the veins are prominent on the upper abdomen, as well as the chest, and flow is usually downwards. In portal vein obstruction the flow is in the normal direction but veins are usually on the lateral wall or, more rarely, radiating from the umbilicus.

A 5.3   Barbiturate overdose.

Bullae appear on areas of pressure in about 6 per cent of patients who develop barbiturate-induced coma. These lesions invariably appear within 24 hours of ingestion of the drug.

A 5.4   (a) Left side of the pons.

(b) Left lateral rectus palsy.

An upper motor neuron lesion of the facial nerve spares the frontalis and/or orbicularis oculi muscles, but may affect the other facial muscles. If the facial palsy is of lower motor neuron type, with failure to wrinkle the forehead or close the eyes tightly, the lesion may occur in the pons, cerebellopontine angle, facial canal, or the face. Pontine lesions giving facial palsy may be associated with ipsilateral sixth cranial nerve palsy and contralateral upper motor neuron hemiplegia. Cerebellopontine angle tumours may involve the fifth (with loss of the corneal reflex), sixth, seventh, and eighth nerves, and may give ipsilateral cerebellar signs and manifestations of increased intracranial pressure. If the lesion is in the facial canal, loss of taste in the anterior two-thirds of the ipsilateral side of the tongue occurs, occasionally associated with hyperacusis from involvement of the stapedius. A facial nerve palsy without other accompanying neurological signs is caused by a lesion distal to the facial canal.

A 5.5   (a) Retroperitoneal fibrosis producing obstructive uropathy and medial displacement of the left ureter.

(b) Methysergide.

(c) Ureterolysis and cessation of drug.

Methysergide, used in the treatment of migraine, may cause retroperitoneal fibrosis. Practolol may cause fibrosis of peritoneum, pleura, and lungs, but not isolated retroperitoneal fibrosis. Retroperitoneal fibrosis is usually suggested by a history of backache, the presence of other fibrosing diseases, evidence of inferior vena caval obstruction, and a high e.s.r. It is confirmed by intravenous or retrograde urography which may show irregular, tapering constrictions and medial displacement of the ureters. Reasonable return of function frequently occurs after ureterolysis.

A 5.6   (a) (i) Heberden's nodes;

(ii) Bouchard's nodes.

(b) Female.

Osteoarthrosis affects the distal interphalangeal joints and is often associated with bony nodules along the joint line (Heberden's nodes) and angulation deformity of the joints. Similar bony nodules may be seen at the proximal interphalangeal joints (Bouchard's nodes). Heberden's and Bouchard's nodes are the result of osteophyte formation at the interphalangeal joints (Fig. 5A, overleaf). The loss of joint space at these joints with soft tissue shadows demonstrating the nodes can be seen on X-ray. Heberden's nodes are more common in women. It is postulated that a single autosomal gene is involved which is dominant in females and recessive in males.

A 5.7   Constrictive pericarditis.

Symptoms and signs suggestive of right-sided heart failure develop in con-

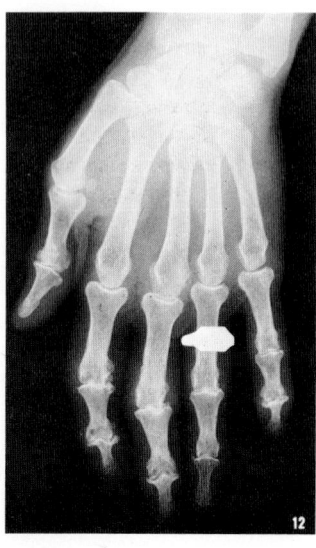

Fig. 5A
Bony nodules at distal interphalangeal joint
(Heberden's nodes) and at proximal inter-
phalangeal joint (Bouchard's nodes).

strictive pericarditis, usually in young or middle-aged adults. The cardiac
origin of the ascites and hepatomegaly is indicated by the marked elevation of
the JVP which has a marked early diastolic collapse (Y descent). Other
confirmatory signs are Kussmaul's sign (paradoxical increase of jugular
venous pressure on inspiration) and pulsus paradoxus. Abdominal swelling
caused by ascites and hepatomegaly usually precedes and overshadows the
peripheral oedema. The absence of orthopnoea is variable and differentiation
from tricuspid stenosis and cardiomyopathies, in which ventricular filling is
impaired, may require further investigation.

A 5.8   (a) Episcleritis.

         (b) Collagen disease, especially rheumatoid arthritis.

Episcleritis is an inflammation that tends to involve the superficial sclera
between the insertion of the rectus muscles and the corneoscleral limbus. It
may occur in isolation, in which case middle-aged men are most frequently
affected, or in patients with collagen disease. In rheumatoid arthritis the sclera
may be affected by (1) episcleritis, (2) necrotizing nodular scleritis, (3)
scleromalacia perforans, and (4) massive granuloma of the sclera.

A 5.9   (a) Nicotinamide;

         (b) (i) Liver;

(ii) lean meat;

(iii) vegetables.

Pellagra in industrialized countries generally occurs in alcoholics whose diets are vitamin- and protein-deficient, leading to niacin and tryptophan deficiency. The early symptoms of pellagra are non-specific but as the vitamin deficiency progresses a sore tongue develops, giving way to severe inflammation of mucous membranes, psychic changes leading to dementia, and dermatitis on areas of skin exposed to the sun. In the acute stage the dermatitis resembles sunburn but with chronicity, skin thickening, scaling, and pigmentation develop. Symmetrical distribution of lesions over sun-exposed areas (Fig. 5B) and over pressure points is characteristic.

Although a diet adequate in niacin and tryptophan and the administration of nicotinamide is the logical treatment, concurrent therapy with thiamin, riboflavin, and pyridoxine should also be given.

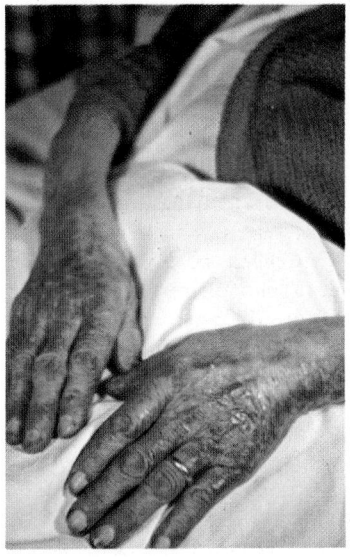

Fig. 5B
Beefy red rash of pellagra on sun-exposed
area of the hands.

A 5.10   (a) Arachnodactyly.

(a) (i) Marfan's syndrome (MS);

(ii) homocystinuria (HC).

Long-surviving patients with HC have some clinical features in common with MS. Arachnodactyly, pectus excavatum or carinatum, long narrow face, lax ligaments, and extopia lentis are common to both. The lens is more likely to be dislocated upwards in MS but downward in HC. The presence of a malar flush, generalized osteoporosis, and mental retardation points to HC, whereas dissecting aneursym of the aorta occurs only in MS. The diagnosis of HC may be confirmed by a positive nitroprusside test for homocystine or by paper electrophoresis of the urine. MS remains a clinical diagnosis. Both are inherited disorders; MS is autosomal dominant with variable penetrance and HC is autosomal recessive.

A 5.11 (a) (i) Keratoderma blenorrhagicum;

(ii) circinate mouth ulceration.

(b) (i) Urethritis and circinate balinitis;

(ii) conjunctivitis and iritis;

(iii) polyarthropathy and sacroileitis.

Genito-urinary or gastrointestinal symptoms usually precede the ocular or rheumatic features of Reiter's syndrome by several days or a few weeks. In Western Europe and North America most cases are associated with venereal disease, but some may follow bacillary dysentery or Yersinia infection. Most patients are male and there is a strong association with HLA-B27. The development of mucocutaneous lesions leaves no doubt about the diagnosis but in their absence the main diagnostic problem concerns the differentiation of Reiter's syndrome from gonococcal arthritis.

A 5.12 (a) Spider naevi.

(b) (i) Cirrhosis of the liver, especially alcoholic;

(ii) viral hepatitis;

(iii) pregnancy;

(iv) rheumatoid arthritis.

An arterial spider consists of a central arteriole, which may be raised with numerous small vessels radiating from it. Pressure on the central arteriole causes the lesion to blanch and if large enough, pulsation may be seen or even felt. Spiders vary in size and are usually found in the vascular territory of the superior vena cava. A few spiders occur in normal persons but many new ones or increasing size of old ones suggests liver disease.

A 5.13 (a) Bilateral parotid gland enlargement.

(b) (i) Sarcoidosis;

       (ii) tuberculosis;

       (iii) white cell neoplasia.

Mikulicz's syndrome consists of parotid swelling and fever, often accompanied by lacrimal adenitis and uveitis. In addition to sarcoidosis it occurs in tuberculosis, leukaemia, Hodgkin's disease, and lupus erythematosus. Uveoparotid fever, or Herrfordt's syndrome, is seen in some patients with sarcoidosis and comprises parotid gland enlargement, anterior uveitis, facial palsy, and fever (which is not usually a feature of sarcoidosis).

    Bilateral painless parotid swelling unassociated with fever may also be seen in patients with cirrhosis, chronic alcoholism, and malnutrition.

A 5.14   (a) Rickets.

       (b) (i) Inadequate diet with little exposure to sunlight;

          (ii) malabsorption;

          (iii) renal disease.

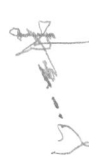

Rickets refers to a number of vitamin D deficiency syndromes occurring in childhood characterized by severe bone pain and periarticular pain, skeletal deformity, growth retardation, depressed plasma Ca $\times$ P ion product, wide osteoid seams in bone, and abnormal proliferation and maturation of the epiphyseal growth plate.

    Severe rickets has a rarely seen, though characteristic, clinical picture of thick skull bones, with prominence of frontal and parietal sutures and rachitic rosary. The latter is produced by swelling of the rachitic intermediate zone at the junction of the costal cartilage and the calcified portion of the rib. The lower portion of the rib cage may be flared out and 'Harrison's groove' produced by the pull of the diaphragm on the yielding rib structure. The deformities of the long bones start as knobbing and prominence of the epiphyses, particularly at the wrists and ankles. Bowing and genu vulgus or varus deformity may subsequently develop.

A 5.15   (a) Exophthalmos.

       (b) Graves' disease.

       (c) (i) Orbital tumour;

          (ii) sphenoid ridge meningioma;

          (iii) thrombosis of the cavernous sinus.

In patients with hyperthyroidism, mild lid retraction and stare are the result of sympathetic overactivity but the remaining abnormalities of Graves' ophthalmopathy such as proptosis, extra-ocular muscle dysfunction, and chemosis, appear to be due to infiltration of the retro-orbital tissues, extra-ocular muscles, and lacrimal gland by lymphocytes, plasma cells, and polymorphonuclear leucocytes, as well as an increase in tissue water, mucopolysaccharides, and mucoproteins.

Although there is usually little diagnostic confusion exophthalmos may also occur in Cushing's syndrome, Turner's syndrome, and cirrhosis. Unilateral exophthalmos should stimulate consideration of orbital tumour, sphenoid ridge meningioma, or thrombosis of the cavernous sinus in reaching a diagnosis.

A 5.16   (a)   Lichen planus of skin and nails.

         (b)   Average duration is 15–24 months, but it may persist for years.

Lichen planus begins with the progressive appearance of intensely pruritic, discrete, shiny, violet, flat-topped, polygonal papules, the flat surface of which reveals pathognomonic grey lines (Wickham's striae). The papules may become confluent as their numbers increase. They may have a symmetrical distribution, the sites of predilection being the flexor surfaces of wrists, forearms, ankles, and abdomen. Papules are rarely seen on the palms and soles. At the site of skin damage, such as a scratch, a linear eruption of lichen planus papules may develop (Koebner's phenomenon). Grey lacy-looking patches are present on the buccal mucosa, tongue, and lips in about 60 per cent of cases with skin involvement. The nails may be involved in one-tenth of cases, with progressive thinning and an increase in longitudinal ridging. Rarely, nails may be completely shed.

A 5.17   (a)   (i)   Vasculitis;

             (ii)   vascular insufficiency of medial soles.

         (b)   (i)   Polyarteritis;

             (ii)   glomerulitis

Although disease of a single organ system may occur in polyarteritis nodosa the patient more often seems to be suffering from a subacute bacterial illness. Peripheral neuritis with severe lower limb pain is common. Then careful search for cutaneous nodules and repeated attempts to confirm the diagnosis by biopsy are necessary. Renal biopsy often shows glomerular disease but is rarely diagnostic and liver biopsy is very unlikely to show the vascular lesion of polyarteritis. Therefore a biopsy, whenever possible, should be obtained from a skeletal muscle exhibiting pain and tenderness. The incidence of renal involvement is very high and is the cause of death in two-thirds of patients with primary polyarteritis.

Pathologically, there are three major types of renal lesions:

1. Polyarteritis with infarction of the kidney. An acute inflammatory infiltration starts in the media but extends to the adventitia and to the intima, inducing thrombosis of the lumen and aneurysm formation.

2. A specific diffuse glomerulitis characterized by capillary microthrombi, focal fibrinoid necroses, polymorph infiltration with crescent formation.

3. Focal glomerulitis with proliferation of the epithelial cells of the capillary tufts, affecting some of the glomeruli.

A 5.18　(a)　Left parotid enlargement.

　　　　　(b)　Acute parotitis.

A parotid swelling is situated mainly in front of the tragus of the pinna, and obliterates the depression normally visible below and in front of the lobule of the ear. Parotid enlargement may occur in debilitated or comatose patients and then suppuration, usually unilateral, often develops. Other causes of unilateral parotid swelling include mumps, blockage of parotid by a calculus, sarcoidosis, tuberculosis, syphilis, lymphadenoma, leukaemia, and mixed cell tumour.

A 5.19　(a)　Purpura.

　　　　　(b)　Henoch–Schönlein purpura.

Renal involvement in Henoch–Schönlein purpura is variable. Although patients may have no signs or symptoms of renal disease at the height of the anaphylactoid purpura, there is usually haematuria or proteinuria. If the disease does not remit spontaneously, hypertensive renal failure may develop. Nephrotic syndrome most commonly affects the 14–18-year age group. Renal disease with skin purpura may also be caused by the haemolytic uraemic syndrome, thrombotic thrombocytopaenic purpura, infective endocarditis, septicaemia, connective tissue disease, and drugs.

A 5.20　(a)　Dystonia of intrinsic muscles of hand;

　　　　　(b)　Drug-induced tardive dyskinaesia.

Neuroleptic (particularly phenothiazines and butyrophenones) and other drugs may provoke acute dystonic reactions in a minority of sensitive individuals. Tardive dyskinaesia occurs after months or years of treatment, usually in the elderly. The typical orofacial movements are often accompanied by chorea of the digits and dystonic spasms of the trunk. Initially, these muscle spasms may occur only on certain actions, such that on writing the arm becomes extended and hyperpronated, and the wrist flexed with fingers extended.

References

GENERAL

Advanced Medicine. Annual reviews of growing points in medicine. Pitman, London.
Beeson, P. B. *et al.* (Ed.) (1979). *Cecil's Textbook of medicine* (15th edn). Saunders, Philadelphia.
Bodley Scott, R. (Ed.) (1978). *Price's Textbook of the practice of medicine* (12th edn). Oxford University Press.
Isselbacher, K. J. *et al.* (Ed.) (1980). *Harrison's Principles and practice of internal medicine* (9th edn). McGraw-Hill, New York.
Medicine. The monthly add-on journal, 2nd and 3rd series. Medical Education (International) Ltd, Oxford.
Papworth, M. H. (1978). *A primer of medicine* (4th edn). Butterworths, London.

CARDIOLOGY

Julian, D. G. (1978). *Cardiology*. Baillière Tindall, London.
Oram, S. (1971). *Clinical heart disease*. Heinemann, London.
van der Werf, T. (1980) *Cardiovascular pathophysiology*. Oxford University Press.

DERMATOLOGY

Shuster, S. (1978). *Dermatology in internal medicine*. Oxford University Press.
Stewart, N. D., Danto, J. L., and Maddin, S. (1974). *Dermatology. Diagnosis and treatment of cutaneous disorders* (3rd edn). Mosby, Saint Louis, Missouri.

ENDOCRINOLOGY

Hall, R. *et al.* (Ed.) (1974). *Fundamentals of clinical endocrinology*. Pitman, London.

GASTROENTEROLOGY

Brooks, F. B. (1978). *Gastrointestinal pathophysiology*. Oxford University Press.
Sherlock, S. (1975). *Diseases of the liver and biliary system* (5th edn). Blackwell, Oxford.
Sleisenger, M. H. and Fordtran, J. S. (1973). *Gastrointestinal disease. Pathophysiology, diagnosis, management*. Saunders, Philadelphia.
Wright, R., Alberti, K. G. M. M., Kerran, S., and Milward-Sadler, G. H. (1979). *Liver and biliary disease*. Saunders, London.

HAEMATOLOGY

de Gruchy, G. C. (1978). *Clinical haematology in medical practice* (4th edn). Blackwell, Oxford.

NEPHROLOGY

Black, D. and Jones, N. F. (1979). *Renal disease* (4th edn). Blackwell, Oxford. (Also 3rd edn, 1972.)

de Wardener, H. E. (1973). *The kidney. An outline of normal and abnormal structure and function* (4th edn). Churchill Livingstone, London.

Leaf, A. and Cotran, R. (1980) *Renal pathophysiology* (2nd edn). Oxford University Press.

NEUROLOGY

Bannister, R. (1978). *Brain's Clinical neurology* (5th edn). Oxford University Press.

Matthews, W. B. and Miller, H. (1979). *Diseases of the nervous system* (3rd edn). Blackwell, Oxford.

OPHTHALMOLOGY

Newell, F. W. (1974). *Ophthalmology: principles and concepts* (3rd edn). Mosby, Saint Louis, Missouri.

RESPIRATORY DISEASE

Crofton, J. and Douglas, A. (1975). *Respiratory diseases* (2nd edn). Blackwell, Oxford.

RHEUMATOLOGY

Hughes, G. R. V. (1977). *Connective tissue diseases*. Blackwell, Oxford.

Subject index

The bold references are to question numbers, not page numbers